Intermittent Fasting for Women

An Essential Guide to Weight Loss, Fat-Burning, and Healing Your Body Without Sacrificing All Your Favorite Foods

© **Copyright 2019**

All Rights Reserved. No part of this book may be reproduced in any form without permission in writing from the author. Reviewers may quote brief passages in reviews.

Disclaimer: No part of this publication may be reproduced or transmitted in any form or by any means, mechanical or electronic, including photocopying or recording, or by any information storage and retrieval system, or transmitted by email without permission in writing from the publisher.

While all attempts have been made to verify the information provided in this publication, neither the author nor the publisher assumes any responsibility for errors, omissions or contrary interpretations of the subject matter herein.

This book is for entertainment purposes only. The views expressed are those of the author alone, and should not be taken as expert instruction or commands. The reader is responsible for his or her own actions.

Adherence to all applicable laws and regulations, including international, federal, state and local laws governing professional licensing, business practices, advertising and all other aspects of doing business in the US, Canada, UK or any other jurisdiction is the sole responsibility of the purchaser or reader.

Neither the author nor the publisher assumes any responsibility or liability whatsoever on the behalf of the purchaser or reader of these materials. Any perceived slight of any individual or organization is purely unintentional.

Contents

INTRODUCTION 1
CHAPTER 1: WHAT IS INTERMITTENT FASTING? 6
CHAPTER 2: SCIENTIFIC BENEFITS OF INTERMITTENT FASTING .12
    INTERMITTENT FASTING: WOMEN VERSUS MEN 16
CHAPTER 3: HOW FASTING IMPACTS WEIGHT LOSS 20
    KETOSIS 24
CHAPTER 4: DIFFERENT INTERMITTENT FASTING TECHNIQUES .27
    THE 16/8 METHOD 28
    THE 5/2 DIET METHOD 29
    THE EAT STOP EAT METHOD 29
    THE ALTERNATING DAY METHOD 30
    THE WARRIOR METHOD 30
    THE SPONTANEITY METHOD 31
    CUSTOMIZATION TECHNIQUES 31
CHAPTER 5: FASTING AND EXERCISE MYTHS EXPLAINED 35
    INTERMITTENT FASTING WILL SLOW YOUR METABOLISM 36
    BY JUST FASTING YOU WILL LOSE WEIGHT 36
    YOU CAN EAT ANYTHING YOU WANT IN BETWEEN FASTS 36
    INTERMITTENT FASTING IS EFFECTIVE AND EVERYONE SEES RESULTS 37
    FASTING IS STARVING YOURSELF AND UNHEALTHY 37
    FASTING LEADS TO MUSCLE LOSS 37

EXERCISING LEADS TO WEIGHT LOSS 38
THE BEST TIME TO EXERCISE IS IN THE MORNING 38
EXERCISE BENEFITS ONLY THE PHYSICAL 38
FASTED WORKOUTS 38
- ☐ *Yoga* *40*
- ☐ *Tai Chi* *41*
- ☐ *Jogging* *41*
- ☐ *Cardio* *41*
- ☐ *Pilates* *42*
- ☐ *Hiking* *42*

CHAPTER 6: BEST FOODS FOR FASTING **43**
LEAFY GREENS 45
GARLIC 46
POTATOES 46
TOMATOES 46
BROCCOLI 46
CAULIFLOWER 46
SUNFLOWER SEEDS 47
ALMONDS 47
BLUEBERRIES 47
RASPBERRIES 47
CHOCOLATE 47
BEANS 48
RICE 48
TOFU 48
SALMON 48
SHELLFISH 48
MEAL PREPPING 49
NOTABLE DIETS 56

CHAPTER 7: GETTING STARTED 62

CHAPTER 8: ONE WEEK STEP-BY-STEP GUIDE 66

   THE 16/8 METHOD 67

      Guideline: 67

      Sunday 68

      Key Points: 68

      Monday (Day 1) 68

      Tuesday (Day 2) 69

      Wednesday (Day 3) 70

      Thursday (Day 4) 71

      Friday (Day 5) 71

      Saturday (Day 6) 72

      Sunday (Day 7) 73

   THE 5/2 METHOD 73

      Sunday 74

      Monday (Day 1) 74

      Tuesday (Day 2) 75

      Wednesday (Day 3) 76

      Thursday (Day 4) 76

      Friday (Day 5) 76

      Saturday (Day 6) 77

      Sunday (Day 7) 77

   THE EAT STOP EAT METHOD 77

      Sunday 78

      Monday (Day 1) 79

      Tuesday (Day 2) 79

      Wednesday (Day 3) 80

      Thursday (Day 4) 80

      Friday (Day 5) 80

- *Saturday (Day 6) 81*
- *Sunday (Day 7) 81*
- *Added Notes on the Eat Stop Eat Method 81*
- ALTERNATE DAY METHOD 81
  - *Sunday 82*
  - *Monday (Day 1) 82*
  - *Tuesday (Day 2) 83*
  - *Wednesday (Day 3) 83*
  - *Thursday (Day 4) 84*
  - *Friday (Day 5) 84*
  - *Saturday (Day 6) 84*
  - *Sunday (Day 7) 84*
- WARRIOR METHOD 85
  - *Sunday 85*
  - *Monday (Day 1) 86*
  - *Tuesday (Day 2) 87*
  - *Wednesday (Day 3) 87*
  - *Thursday (Day 4) 88*
  - *Friday (Day 5) 88*
  - *Saturday (Day 6) 88*
  - *Sunday (Day 7) 89*
- SPONTANEITY METHOD 89

CHAPTER 9: DOS AND DON'TS OF INTERMITTENT FASTING 92
CONCLUSION 97
CHECK OUT MORE BOOKS BY ELIZABETH MOORE 99

Introduction

This book is dedicated to the individual who wishes to improve her life through the transformative practice of Intermittent Fasting and weight loss. We will explore and discover what it takes to truly transform our day-to-day life into a positive and beneficial lifestyle, not only by simply cutting out some meals here and there but also by taking time to examine our habits, analyze our life choices up to this point, and be truthful with ourselves about our bodies and minds. This is not a casual diet fad manifesto but an immersive guideline to successful and safe weight loss. What it takes to cut weight and keep it off does not have to involve quitting your favorite foods and guilty pleasures, although it will require discipline, confidence, and a true desire to transform your life for the better. This well-rounded book is not a miracle cure for problems but a book that presents methods to transform your body and mindset. Your outlook on life is just as important as physical health, and here, we will explore the relationship between the two.

Transformation is the most important word in this book. We will aim to keep transformation as the key goal – not only the transformation of our diet or health but a transformation of our entire lives. If this seems too far out of reach, do not be discouraged – it is easier than you think. Transformation does not require us to change who we truly are. We can keep all the things we love, but it will require a rewiring of how we view ourselves and the world around us. What could normally trigger a negative or detrimental attitude will be altered and viewed from a different perspective, a perspective that comes from a place of self-love and confidence. By applying the knowledge and practices we are about to learn into our lives, we can develop a lifestyle that will become second nature and only help us stay healthful physically and mentally.

In the chapters to come, we will discuss the ins and outs of Intermittent Fasting with an emphasis on women's weight loss in today's busy and complicated world. Women have had to battle more difficulties than men for all of written history, and today is no different. Naturally, the extra stress on women to look and behave a certain way makes it very difficult to maintain balance during the mundane day-to-day tasks, thus making healthful lifestyles a choice that is overlooked or flat out cannot be obtained. All the fad diets and exercise cannot extinguish centuries of struggle, no, but taking care of our bodies on an individual level while navigating the tough social terrain is a step in the right direction to health and happiness. No technology or wonder drug will ever be the miracle cure it's claiming to be, but creating a wonderful life and feeling amazing doesn't have to be difficult. In fact, the path to balanced health comes with a few simple changes in the way we treat food and ourselves. We need to reevaluate the social norms and their detrimental effect on our lifestyles. We need to filter out the noise of our fast-paced lifestyles and redesign our eating habits to benefit each of us as an individual. There is no end all be all solution to great health; our bodies and our world are constantly changing, and we need to change with it.

With the advent of modified foods and advanced science, our current society seems to work efficiently. Our technological progress has provided luxuries beyond the fantasies of the population that thrived only a couple of hundred years ago, but there are still problems pertaining to the influence on our health with these advancements. Travel technology, accompanied by a globe completely interconnected by the Internet, has allowed cultures to cross-pollinate. Rich foods from all around the world are accessible for the first time, but so is overconsumption. The luxuries of fast food and processed snacks have paved the way for our society of diversity and information to turn to quick satisfaction rather than mindful consumption, this inevitably turning into a weight gain problem in our society.

As services and goods become easier to acquire, less emphasis and attention is given to our bodies and minds. We replace healthful lifestyles with the laziest ones. Food becomes simply something we "drive-thru" a tiny window for, time set aside for exercise takes a back seat to social media, and instead of mindfulness, we find ourselves zombie-like and nullified. Obesity and excessive weight gain are abundant, and confidence in ourselves seems to be at an all-time low. As the current structure slips away into a health crisis, there are things that individuals can do to counteract the negative effects, no matter how lazy you are.

This is where Intermittent Fasting (IF) comes into play. Although a practice used regularly by ancient cultures and indigenous ones today, fasting has become much more popular in contemporary culture in recent years. Fasting is the intentional cutting off of caloric intake to benefit the body and mind. Intermittent Fasting is cutting off caloric intake for a predetermined set part of the day – that is, only eating for a respected window of hours. Not eating throughout the day may sound like no fun at first, and the mere thought of the starving feeling is discomforting, and it may be, at first, but through a dedicated practice of Intermittent Fasting, we give rise to a new feeling, one of empowerment and control. Many were raised to believe that the ideal diet is having three square meals a day and plenty of snacks in between, but the science and visible results prevail as our society embraces the practice and fasting finds its way into our daily lives.

Intermittent Fasting is a simple and very effective way not only to lose weight safely and naturally but also keeps the mind sharp by creating a distinct awareness of the food we take for granted every day. By cutting caloric intake for certain times of the day, we find a more structured eating plan, one that the body benefits from as you cut unnecessary weight while also benefitting the brain by changing the way we look at meals. These benefits balance the mind-body experience, building new relationships with food, health, and ourselves. The balance of body and mind is the best preventative measure to ensure that we feel amazing every day, awake refreshed, and live our lives to the fullest.

If you are reading this, you've no doubt tried many other techniques to lose weight and feel great. If you have been frightened away from fasting because it's been presented as extreme or unhealthy, do not worry. In this book, we will focus on the key elements of Intermittent Fasting and how it can help women lose weight while not changing their lives completely. In the chapters to come, we will focus heavily on Intermittent Fasting as a path to transformation of the body and mind. The reason we choose to view this as a transformative practice is simple: we want to treat ourselves not as only scientific explanations and results but as powerful beings that are capable of taking control of their lives and transforming them. When seeing our bodies through this lens, we can visualize the results of our practice, motivating ourselves to achieve these goals. Mindfulness and awareness are key components to weight loss and an amazing life in general.

In this book, we aim to present methods of fasting that can be easily customized to fit your schedule. We will explore the science and safety of Intermittent Fasting, suitable foods, and dietary guidelines, and how safely to exercise while fasting. This is a transformational path not only of the body but of the mind and perception of health.

You may not have discovered the right material that presents the practice in an appealing way, but rest assured that this book is for you. Let's begin this journey with an open mind and open heart as we introduce Intermittent Fasting to our lives.

Chapter 1: What is Intermittent Fasting?

Let's get right to the point. Fasting is a relatively simple practice that yields incredible and complicated results. The effects that fasting has on the body and mind seem unfathomable: weight loss, blood sugar regulation, blood pressure regulation, and growth hormone regulation – only to name a few important ones. In recent years, science has come full force to support these claims, not to mention the thousands of videos online of people's results now that fasting has hit the mainstream. There are different types of fasting as well as many ways to fast.

Within the abundant array of different methods and individual changes any one person may implement, there is a wealth of potential ways to impact the health of the body and mind in positive ways. Fasting, in a general and broad definition, is the practice of willingly abstaining from something, usually food and drink. Whether it is simply not eating chocolate for a week or two or even cutting out all solid foods for a month, no matter how large or small the impact the abstinence has on you, that is fasting from your chosen food. Another more intensive fast would be dry fasting. Dry fasting is the complete abstinence from every source of solid or liquid food for any predetermined period, and, of course, willingly. Although not completely out of the question for beginners, these styles of fasting are used more sparingly than the style we aim to focus on, and that practice is called Intermittent Fasting or IF for short.

IF is very similar to the practices described above, but instead of completely fasting for days at a time, you would choose a certain time of the day, say an eight-hour period. This time window would be the only time you ingest foods as much as you'd like depending on your personal goals. There may also be other rules you set yourself, but there's more on customizing your practice later in the book. The idea of intentionally choosing not to eat may be contradictory to many of the views on food that our culture holds dear. Abundance and indulgence run rampant in our world, and the more you have, the better, right? Not so much. As we now see the results of the destructive habits we have formed, we must look to other answers, better practices, and mindful analyzation of what and when we eat. Changing our eating habit is no small feat; it takes a strong will and a desire to attain a more meaningful and healthy life, one that is not overburdened with sugary snacks and stress caused by overeating. As we can see, IF is not so much a new fad diet but a distinct and progressive lifestyle choice. And although these practices have only recently hit the mainstream in our world today, there is a long and fruitful lineage of practices from cultures all around the world that practiced fasting, and we look to these cultures and our distant ancestors for inspiration and guidance on this journey.

Before today's fast-paced society took hold of our diets, fasting played a very important role in essentially every culture and society around the world. Whether it was for spiritual purposes, health reasons, or some intense ritual, fasting was a lynchpin in many lifestyles throughout human history. Even before humans had science to explore the details of how our bodies work on a microscopic level, we knew that fasting was a source of good health and wellbeing. Primitive cultures would often require fasting before battles and even as an initiatory milestone during puberty. The prehistorical humans surely weren't as concerned about their weight and appearances as we are now, but the hunter-gatherer lifestyle would seemingly fit nicely within the scope of IF. Wandering place to place in search of nutrients, there may have been plenty of time in between meals, but is this fasting? Sure, the ancient tribes probably went long periods without food but probably not willingly. It's impossible to truly find out what the ancient cultures were thinking and practicing, but here, we see potential caloric restriction that influenced early man in incredible ways, perhaps even influencing the onset of agriculture and settling.

As humans progressed and began settling, we see a more prominent and definitive practice of fasting. We see all the big hitters in the religious world advocating for it; Jesus Christ, Muhammed, and Buddha all viewed fasting as a purification process. Commonly based on religious grounds, fasting became a practice of sacrifice, giving up something to show a respected god or entity that you were devoted and deserved good graces from powerful beings. The idea of giving up something so precious, which was required to survive, would surely appease the gods. Certainly, as these practices caught on, the humans, religious or not, felt the results of their fasts. Fasting stays a prominent aspect of medicine as the timeline progresses onward into some ancient cultures that we have better historical documentation of.

The ancient Greek philosophers valued fasting among their other important contributions to our current world. Hippocrates, the father of modern medicine, focused heavily on fasting for a balanced and healthful life. He spoke and promoted the practice while also prescribing it to his patients. The Greek philosophy drew heavily from nature; the observation that humans lose their appetite when they are sick showed the Greek philosophers and doctors that the body naturally restricts caloric intake when ill, and thus there must be some value to the healing potential of willingly abstaining from caloric intake. Another father of contemporary medicine who advocated for fasting was Paracelsus, the inventor of toxicology. He wrote, "Fasting is the greatest remedy, the physician within." The reference to "the physician within" alludes to the body having a natural ability to intuitively heal itself, let alone have assistance by the human mind through the willingness to abstain and attention to the nuances of the mind-body connection. These ancient ideas helped build the foundation of our current state of medicine, but perhaps we need to return to the ideas held dear to our ancestors.

While considering that our ancient ancestors and some of the most prominent minds of our time utilized IF as a means of attaining optimal health, we look forward to today's world. Although the Western world relies heavily on processed foods and a constant intake of foods throughout the day, many contemporary societies live quite the opposite and thrive just as well or even better. One example that stands out is the Hunzakuts of Northern Pakistan. Thriving in the Hunza valley, these people are well known to live well past one hundred years of age, even documenting one woman who was 130 years old! Along with this incredible longevity, the Hunza are living without hardly any degenerative disease. With their diets being high in mineral content and low in sodium, their longevity can be attributed to this, but there is another key factor that suits our purposes. The Hunza people have a very limited food intake. Even without the complicated science and meal plans, they have withheld a standard of longevity quite naturally. Their recent history before being touched by civilization had very interesting patterns that they adhered to not out of choice but simply because that was how they lived their lives. The Hunza people's annual harvest each year would be exhausted, and they would live with minimal caloric intake for weeks at a time each spring. Once the last year's food supply was depleted, they would have minimal sustenance until the new harvest began. With more modern science showing that limited caloric intake has amazing effects on the body and brain, as we will explore, the longevity of the Hunza is linked to their IF lifestyle, along with their distinct diet.

So, around the world, we see fasting being used for survival and necessity, but what about fasting for other purposes? IF finds itself permeating so many aspects of our culture that it cannot be ignored as a key element in human life and survival.

Today, we see fasting prominent in the most widely practiced religions. These holidays and traditions permeate all of the cultures in our interconnected world. Ramadan is a holy month in Islamic religions, during the ninth month of their calendar adherents fast from dawn to dusk – this is IF at its core. Christianity has its holy fast called Lent. This six-week period begins on Ash Wednesday and ends on Easter Sunday, where during this time, there are many celebrations and practices, but fasting remains a very important aspect. For Jewish cultures, Yom Kippur stands out as an important fast day, comprised of a 25-hour fast and intensive prayer. These examples being the most popular, let's not forget that all religions and cultures use fasting. The non-religious and more fact-based mind benefit from fasting's rigorous power to change and alter health. Mahatma Gandhi famously undertook seventeen fasts while fighting for India's independence, showing that fasting isn't simply for health or religious benefit, but can be used to usher in revolution and political change. However, what about all of us who aren't religious adherents or world-changing revolutionaries?

The history of fasting lays a solid foundation that cannot be ignored in modern times. New science technology is confirming the history and reassuring contemporary populations that IF is a safe, effective, and simple path to overall health. Not only is fasting resting comfortably on the shoulders of science and history, but it also has perks in the consumerist world we live in. Since fasting requires no prescriptions, no fitness contraptions, and no expensive supplements, the practice fits nicely within our money-hungry, materialist society. Simply abstaining from something you love to eat for a day or two changes your outlook on your potential to take control of your life and literally will save you money as you will be consuming less than usual. As practical as it sounds, many feel that it is too good to be true, that simply not eating could not possibly affect the body and brain as much as people claim. And sure, at first glance, it seems like a gimmick that celebrity doctors want to scam you with, but given the test of time and solid science, fasting will remain a pivotal practice in the rearranging of our lives in the Western world, an action that desperately needs to be put into play.

Now that we've gotten acquainted with the history and basics of fasting and its role in our society let's focus on some in-depth science on IF to truly grasp what will happen when we begin this amazing journey of transformation.

Chapter 2: Scientific Benefits of Intermittent Fasting

Relying on the knowledge of ancient cultures grants a certain amount of philosophical insight but is limited in the scientific background our twenty-first-century minds require to be rest assured. Fortunately, many studies on IF are popping up all over the Internet, with sound scientific evidence that fasting is as safe and effective, if not more so than any other diet that hits the mainstream. For decades, we have thought that what we eat is the most important aspect of whether or not our diets are considered healthy. However, many other factors are in play. Not only what we eat, but how it's prepared, where it's sourced, and when we eat. These combined with physical and mental exercise create our state of health, and IF affects all of these aspects.

By taking on an IF routine, we funnel our view of food and meals through a new lens, thus transforming our mindset about food and the food we ingest and when. This transformation has been shown to increase self-worth, while simultaneously reduce stress, which on a psychological level is incredibly beneficial for someone looking to lose weight. Let's keep this positive outlook and confidence in mind as we approach IF from a strictly scientific perspective.

In a very broad sense, IF's physical results are attributed to calorie restriction. It makes sense, right? Eat less, get thin. But it goes deeper than this simple equation. Lab studies have shown that calorie restriction has been attributed to the reduction of illnesses related to death and lengthened lifespans. Studies have shown that in mice obesity, the risk of metabolic diseases are lowered due to caloric restriction – these reactions having been also proven to translate to humans. Not only can the restrictions help prevent obesity, but they were also shown to reset circadian rhythms and balance the rhythm of hormonal secretions. These rhythms, of which there are many, keep our body in check, ensuring that our body is running smoothly and efficiently. This biological rhythm is very apparent when a fast begins. The rhythm of your digestive system becomes very clear while fasting. Since digestion is essentially 'turned off' once we go to bed, it is subsequently turned back on the moment we intake calories the next morning. So, if we restrict calorie intake, our digestive system will rest until we eat again; while it rests, it repairs itself. By giving our systems plenty of time to repair in between meals, we achieve a simple yet effective and concise practice that assists our body with its natural healing methods. With IF and assigning a strict consumption window, we can actively engage with our natural digestive rhythm, keeping it in sync with the rest of our body as we see fit. The digestive system seems to be an obvious player in weight loss, but what about the control center and epic organ, the human brain?

The human brain is mysterious and complicated; science has certainly only scratched the surface of what must be an infinite amount of investigation into the brain. As the 'control center' of our entire body, it plays a major role in weight loss. The brain not only influences the physical aspects of the body, hormone regulation, and autonomous actions like breathing and blood pumping, but also more in-depth metaphysical ideas, like thought and emotion, are considered to be housed in the brain to some extent. As mysterious as it is, we will stand with these claims. And so, our ideas will play a huge role in our IF journey, and a positive outlook and practicing confidence-building affirmations will go hand in hand with the fasting experience. So consider the brain an avenue for thought and emotion. You are in control and IF will help you come to this realization.

We've spent our whole lives thinking and believing that the societal structure of diets and foods are the most efficient. We need to break from these patterns and do what is best for us individually. Again, no one way of living will work for everyone. On the scientific level, we send signals to our brain that allow it to regulate and restore where need be. So, naturally, if you were to eat less or not eat when you normally do, the brain will assume that the food is scarce and will take the necessary actions. Although the brain may reduce the metabolic rate and attempt to conserve fat reserves, it is still burning reserved fat instead of recently ingested sugars, combined with suitable exercise (found later in the book). This is a very effective and safe weight loss strategy. However, let's not forget that the brain will also start releasing growth hormones to regulate and account for new changes in diet and routine. These are hormones that have been shown to increase longevity and reduce the effects of aging. The brain isn't the only organ that responds positively to IF though.

Many wonder about the idea of the heart being the center of love and emotion. The symbolic idea of the heart is timeless, but what role can it play in our IF journey? The heart regulates blood flow, then the blood distributes nutrients and antibodies to all parts of the body. Considering the major causes of heart disease – cholesterol, blood pressure, weight, and diabetes – we find studies that show how IF assists in balancing all these bodily functions. The influence that this kind of fasting can have on these functions is important. As mentioned before, IF can help reset and assist the body to heal naturally. So, in turn, fasting helps regulate and balance these functions, then fasting directly influences the heart and its major enemies. We will discuss later in the book the potential risks of fasting, but here, we would like to state that some cases have found that extensive fasting can be attributed to electrolyte imbalances, which could affect the heart in negative ways.

The third major organ we want to focus on is the liver. The liver acts as a filtration system for the body while also producing bile to be sent to the intestines. As the filtration system, the liver will play a key role in the positive effects of IF. The caloric restriction itself acts as a symbolic representation of purification while quite literally not consuming any foods for a prolonged period will assist the liver in repairing itself. One particular study also shows us that when calories are restricted, the liver secretes a protein that adjusts the liver's metabolism. The regulation of the metabolism is key in producing weight loss results, and as we've seen, fasting interacts with the metabolism on many levels.

The science that has dedicated itself to fasting has shown what many believed for centuries before computers – that fasting is an all-around beneficial practice for overall wellbeing. Along with the three major organs discussed above, some key points should be emphasized:

- It gives the body more energy by assisting in the creation of mitochondria, which are power sources within every cell of your body. This gives you the energy that is used throughout the body. Having more energy will only assist in keeping up regular exercise and daily duties.
- It boosts growth hormone secretions in the brain. Although available in supplements, wouldn't human growth hormones (HGH) be more effective naturally occurring in the brain? By fasting, we increase the levels secreted by the brain, thus taking advantage of the hormone's natural ability to slow the effects of aging, improve cognitive performance, and protect the brain's health overall.

- It and its caloric restrictions allow the body to burn up stored fat rather than sugars. Fat is a cleaner source of energy than carbs or sugars and reduces inflammation by lowering free radical production, and free radicals are thought to oxidize cells which could lead to autoimmune diseases and the like.
- It reduces inflammation which is attributed to many common diseases, such as dementia and obesity. Inflammation damages cells and IF helps to clean away the damaged cells. Ketones are produced through the burning of fat instead of sugar, and they regulate inflammation. IF also helps the body not become resistant to insulin. Insulin can potentially build up in the blood and create inflammation.

With the incredible effects that IF presents, it is no wonder that it was common amongst our ancestors and now common in the mainstream during the twenty-first century. We know through this science that IF can help us on so many levels, but what about our main goal with this book – weight loss? If we are to focus on shedding some pounds, we need to look deeper into the specific effects that this kind of fasting has on our excess fat and body image as a whole.

Intermittent Fasting: Women Versus Men

There is much debate about the different effects that IF has on women versus the effects that men experience. Although quite similar in many ways, there are distinct differences in the chemistry that makes up the different genders. Even when it comes to fasting, women should approach the practice a little differently than men.

Some studies show that low-energy diets can negatively affect fertility in women. The evolutionary nature of the female body to monitor and tune in to any threats to fertility makes the decreased supply of food and nutrients a huge red flag to the intuition of the woman's body. The sensitivity of women's hormonal balance is directly related to caloric intake and energy supply. In the past, body fat percentage was thought to be the key factor when it came to drastic hormonal changes, but now it is understood that energy, in general, plays a huge role as well. As for IF, the hormonal changes are the body's reactions to environmental conditions being altered, as we've discussed, so this combined with women can result in heightened sensitivity to changes.

There have been some documented cases of women missing menstrual cycles, experiencing drastic metabolic disruption, and uncontrollable binge eating during fasting routines. While these experiences are incredibly rare, it's important to take into account that the human body is mysterious, and many people have completely different experiences under very similar circumstances. So when considering an IF routine, we need to take great caution and listen to our bodies closely if we choose to go through with the practice.

What causes such rare side effects stem from the environmental influence that stimulates the hormonal glands in the brain. These glands – hypothalamus, pituitary, and gonadal – work together to regulate hormones that act on the reproductive organs. This leads us to conclude that when the precise and specific cycle needed to regulate the hormones is disrupted, it could have adverse effects. Why this seems to occur more often to women rather than men is unknown. There is speculation about a particular molecule called kisspeptin that may contribute to this phenomenon. Although kisspeptin exists in both male and female bodies, there is much more of it in women. This molecule may be the culprit, but it is until undetermined.

With what we know about the effects on fertility, we need to take into consideration the role that metabolism plays in all this. Metabolism and fertility work together to benefit each other in many ways. So if the hormones are being disrupted, physical reactions in the body can be concerning. Another topic of debate is the fact that women typically consume less protein than men. So, while fasting, there's an intake of less protein, and less protein is going to mean less amino acids, which are needed to stimulate estrogen receptors.

Again, we see the hormonal faculties being potentially disrupted by taking on an IF routine. While we need to keep this in mind, these rare occurrences shouldn't scare you away from fasting completely. However, if you experience any of the following conditions while fasting, you should end the fast as soon as possible. Break your fast if you experience the following:

- Irregular menstrual cycle
- Hair loss
- Wild mood swings
- Noticeable digestive irregularities
- Feeling abnormal and consistent cold
- Extreme intolerance to stress

As we take these potential side effects on IF into consideration, we also need to consider the fact that it is not for everyone. While the practice is very effective for some people, not everyone is going to enjoy fasting, let alone find benefits in the practice if they simply aren't built for it. If you would describe yourself as unhealthy or new to exercise, then fasting should be preceded by dietary changes and casual exercise. This will prepare your body for the fast and act to reduce shock on your body. Any eating disorders should be dealt with extreme care when approaching fasting as well. And, of course, women who are pregnant should not fast at all.

While women need a little more nuance and attention to detail when considering IF compared to men, we need not let this discourage us from our intended goals in this book. If anything, the complexity of the female body should be an attribute we find intriguing and beautiful, rather than assuming women's complexity is a hindrance. The main rule is to listen to your body, be aware of your changes, and build a relationship with your body. If you find that IF is not going to work for you, you can still gain much from this book. Taking the ideas and methods that we will explore in subsequent chapters can be modified to suit any path with a little alteration and thought.

Chapter 3: How Fasting Impacts Weight Loss

We have discussed the science and effects fasting has on your body, but let's take that information and apply it directly to weight loss. We have mentioned weight loss regarding fasting, but how is this put into practice? You cannot simply fast for a week and expect drastic weight loss. However, by keeping fasting a part of our everyday diet, we allow our body to adapt to changes more easily, and thus can implement other practices that go hand in hand with fasting to ensure maximum results. Remember, weight loss is not only attributed to calorie restriction, but definable results are also seen with overall physical and mental health. Let's start with why we want to lose weight in the first place.

Physical appearance plays an integral role in our society. Billboards and commercials fill the air with super skinny models, forcing our minds to think that there is one true way women are supposed to look. This is completely unfair, and it attacks the mind as a whole. In good practice, we should try and avoid these thought patterns as much as possible and focus on our personal goals. Physically appearing attractive does not imply health. Too skinny, too fat –

these words mean nothing if our bodies and minds are not balanced and healthy. So, let's find out why we want to cut weight with a few personal questions to ask ourselves: *Do I simply want to be beautiful? Do I want to lose weight for longevity? Is my body shape hindering me in some way? Do I need to lose weight for health purposes?* Even the healthiest of people will strive for more balance. No attainable end goal applies to everyone. You need to find your ideal goal and go from there. By taking time to contemplate why we want to or need to lose weight, we can hone in on our specific goals and aspire to attain them through specific practices directed at specific results.

Once we find ourselves being truthful with ourselves about body image, we can begin a true weight loss practice and with it a fasting regimen. But how will this fasting help us cut weight? Aside from the science showing us that Intermittent Fasting reduces inflammation, assists in hormone regulation, and burns cleaner energy, we need to view the fast through a psychological lens.

By even thinking about starting an IF routine, you have already started to change your life. The thoughts that cross your mind about wanting something better for yourself is just the beginning of what could become a dramatic life-altering transformation. The desire for longevity and to be healthful are very common goals; unfortunately, many people suppress these desires in exchange for an easier, way less healthy lifestyle. As this downward spiral progresses, one becomes caught in a seemingly endless loop of processed foods, social media, and laziness. By digging ourselves out of the typical routine, we have the opportunity to reinvent ourselves, to break the wicked cycle, and begin a new life. IF is a great place to begin for this process – not only do you break the detrimental meal cycle, but you also begin to see changes in your thought processes about everything else in your life that may be preventing you from living a healthy and happy life. By being persistent and dedicated, we can begin breaking away from the standard lifestyle. By eliminating the unneeded stress, we also assist ourselves in losing our unneeded weight.

The relationship between stress and obesity has been studied extensively, and there is a link between the two. As the obesity rate began to increase quickly in the United States, scientists soon realized that the problem wasn't limited to only wealthy countries but was a global problem. Thought initially to be a product of overeating and lack of exercise, soon studies showed that many other factors contributed to this pressing issue. Obesity-related illnesses have been linked to industrial, cultural, and, of course, genetic predispositions –all being stressors that are out of our control. Our surroundings cause these stressors, and our society plays a huge role in weight management. Stress is a response in our bodies that is critical for survival. The 'flight or fight' response ensured our survival in prehistoric times and allowed us to adapt to our environment. When we are stressed, our autonomic nervous system is activated; this system regulates heart rate, blood pressure, hormone regulation, and digestion. As we see here, these are the same major functions that IF has been shown to help balance and regulate.

Many of the people who have problems with obesity react to stress by eating food. However, this 'comfort' food is not worth the trouble. Much of the comforting food is very high in fats and sugar, not to mention usually consumed outside of the individual's routine. This may serve as a quick fix for stress, but it can lead to addiction-like behavior and overeating. It is no secret that the food that is valued in our culture is not very healthy, and with the advent of GMO foods and soil that is depleted of nutrients from pesticides, even our fruits and vegetable are not up to par. The food problem is a huge issue today, in fact, unavoidable, but there are ways we go about our lives that counteract much of the problem. Eating nutrient-rich foods that are grown locally and avoiding frozen or prepackaged meals will go a long way to reduce stress. We will go into detail about the suitable meals for IF in a later chapter. By being mindful about our relationship with food is only going to help us in our journey to transformation.

Another issue with weight loss is physical activity. Many people feel that they do not have time to exercise or simply have become so out of shape that the idea of exercise never comes to mind: this is unacceptable. Some may hear the word exercise and instantly picture in their minds a sweaty, beefed-up man lifting weights in front of a mirror. This is a very narrow-minded approach to exercise. Instead of these stereotypical ideas of what it takes to be healthy, let's consider less intensive images. Someone in normal everyday clothing walking casually on a trail in the wilderness or perhaps slowly stretching on a yoga mat in a quiet room – this is exercise too. We don't have to hit the gym to have a balanced physical lifestyle, but simply moving around and getting the blood flowing can suffice. Studies have shown that stress is reduced with a casual exercise routine that even in the moments of the stressful situation, a quick stretch or walk around the block will help alleviate the stress. We will discuss the relationship between IF and exercise later.

So, we see that stress is an important aspect of weight management; it affects the very same major functions that IF has been shown to affect. Combined with a more mindful diet, moderate exercise, and truthful self-image, we see the formation of a very safe and effective routine for weight loss. Now, let's look at what is happening to excess fat when we are in the midst of a fast.

As discussed above, we have found that fasting improves health in many ways. The most accepted science on IF states that fasting influences the circadian rhythms and various other systems needed to live. Circadian rhythms are built in biological processes that act like a biological clock, similar to other natural rhythms such as the tides or seasonal rhythms. These rhythms are controlled by the hypothalamus and can be altered and trained from outside influences, such as light, darkness, food, and IF, respectfully. Organs in your body respond to food restriction and can act to reset these rhythms. Food restriction also affects the microbiome of your gut –

all the bacteria and ecosystem of your gut has its own rhythm as well. As your body resets and the energy from your latest meal is used up, the body turns to fat reserves. The fat reserves release fatty acids which find their way to the liver where they are then converted into ketones. The ketones provide energy for muscles and help to prevent disease processes by protecting neurons. Although, if ketone levels become too high, it could be dangerous. This complicated process is the underlying physical benefit of IF: resetting the internal clocks and using fat reserves. The fat reserves having been reduced, we now find ourselves weighing less safely and effectively. When considering this, we need to dig a little deeper into what ketosis is and how it works.

Ketosis

Much information you find online about IF or weight loss leads to websites and articles dedicated to ketosis and keto diets. Although the ketosis diets are not mandatory for IF, it is a good idea to be educated on the process of ketosis itself and how it interplays with IF.

Ketosis pops up a lot in conversations about health and current diet trends; it is one of the more popular diets on the Internet and yields plenty of success stories from people who practice the diet. But what is ketosis exactly? It can be a positive or a negative thing depending on the context and situation. Ketosis is a natural process that occurs in the body as a metabolic process. Similar to what we've discussed, when your body doesn't have any quick energy to burn, such as carbohydrates from a recent meal, it will burn stored fat instead. This process makes ketones. If the ketone levels in the blood get too high, there can be complicated problems – typically insulin and other hormones prevent the ketone levels from getting too high. However, if there are issues with insulin production, this can be an issue. This is why people with diabetes find themselves in an unwanted ketosis state if they're not using enough insulin and often avoid inducing the state intentionally. A healthy normal body that consumes a balanced diet is in control of the amount of fat it burns and typically won't make ketones. Aside from just restricting carbohydrate intake, ketosis can also be induced by pregnancy and long exercise routines. The ketosis state can most certainly be viewed as a survival mechanism built into the human body. When we have no quick energy to use, or we have no food to ingest, our body switches over to creating ketones and using stored fat to power the body. We see here how ketosis fits into our IF lifestyle. If we restrict calories, especially from carbohydrate-rich foods, the ketosis state will take hold, and we can start burning unwanted and excess fat.

As a weight loss strategy, ketosis diets are effective and safe when practiced with attention to our bodies and state of mind. Not unlike a paleo diet or the popular Atkins diet from decades ago, the low-carb strategy can be very beneficial if used wisely. The diet has been shown to assist the body to maintain muscle and make you feel less hungry. Obviously, fasting will induce a ketosis-like state very quickly, but reducing carbohydrate intake to less than 60 grams a day for four to five days can start a ketosis-like state as well. The diet has been implemented to some success for treatment of many serious diseases including epilepsy.

As with any diet, a ketogenic diet needs to be practiced with great care and with meticulous attention to your body's changes. If the ketone levels in your body get too high, they can build up in the blood and ketoacidosis can take hold. Ketoacidosis causes the built-up ketones to turn the blood very acidic and can result in a coma or even death. Ketone levels can be tested in urine or blood, and it is always a good idea to test if you choose to practice a ketogenic diet. Along with unsafe fasting practices, ketoacidosis can be caused by alcoholism, dehydration, and an overactive thyroid. If you are affected by these symptoms, it is best to check with your doctor before attempting any diet or fast that may induce a ketogenic state.

So, not only do we see an IF routine as directly affecting our circadian rhythms and reducing fat, but the practice acts as a building block to other weight loss protocol. Through fasting, we influence the systems of the body that cause stress, while simultaneously taking societal stress off ourselves by developing a better diet and attitude. The IF routine affects our idea of exercise, not only by freeing time to exercise but also by inducing a ketosis-like state and exercising. We burn fat reserves quicker than if we were eating the same foods at the same time. This combination will be the basis of our weight loss regimen. Now, we need to find a fasting technique that is best suited to our needs.

As we continue on our transformative journey, with science in mind, we need to explore the many different ways we can introduce IF into our lives. There is an infinite number of ways to start your IF routine, but we will focus on some of the more prominent methods that have taken the Internet by storm in recent years.

Chapter 4: Different Intermittent Fasting Techniques

Now that we have discussed how your body will react to fasting let's discuss the many different forms of fasting. Although there are seemingly infinite ways to go about your Intermittent Fasting routine, we will focus on six methods that are popular among fitness experts and the fasting community. We will discuss the suitable timing of 'eating windows', the duration of time in the day when you are allowed to eat, and compare each method so you can successfully choose the best one for your lifestyle. Although fasting has its roots in religion and spirituality, we will not go extensively into these practices, but if you wish to combine your spiritual goals with these methods, you can go right ahead.

At this point, we would like to state that keeping a fasting notebook helps immensely for someone just starting out. By recording our experiences and documenting how successful or unsuccessful our routine is, we can find insight into ourselves and also organize the aspects of our routine that may need to be altered or customized. It is not mandatory to have a notebook, but throughout this book, we will be keeping track of our experiences and analyzing our regimen to understand better what works for us as individuals.

As we move on to explore these popular methods, take note of what they entail and which styles pique your interest as you learn about them. The methods we will explore are as follows:
1. The 16/8 Method
2. The 5:2 Method
3. The Eat Stop Eat Method
4. Alternating Day Fasts
5. The Warrior Method
6. The Spontaneity Method

We will also be discussing tips for customizing your routine. The point of this is to personalize your fasting, so it suits you perfectly. This will optimize the results and also allow the practice to become something you created for yourself, which in turn, builds an intimate relationship with your practice promoting dedication and confidence.

The particular method you choose will have a great deal to do with your day-to-day schedule and mindset. Let's choose wisely and give much thought to the various benefits of different methods, but keep in mind the result can be obtained through any of these methods. Let's also be fair in saying that the time windows can be altered to give or take an hour if need be. If one method doesn't quite work for you, do not be disheartened; simply try another method or customize your current choice.

The 16/8 Method

Also known as the Leangain's method, this method was popularized by Martin Berkhan. The eating window for this style is eight hours with a sixteen-hour fasting time. So if you sleep eight hours, awake, then restrict caloric intake for eight hours, then you can eat as much as you like until bedtime. Another example would be to awake, start your eight-hour eating window, then begin fasting for the evening and during sleep. This is a common choice for people who already skip breakfast. Tea and coffee have no calories, so they are still allowed to be consumed, obviously without sugar added.

Overview:
- Sixteen hours of fasting
- Eight-hour consumption window
- Zero-calorie drinks allowed

The 5/2 Diet Method

This method looks more like a diet than a proper fast, but it is a popular method for weight loss and often finds its way into IF circles. First popularized by Michael Mosley, it is also called the 'Fast Diet'. This method involves your normal eating routine for five days of the week then restricting your caloric intake to 600 calories or less for two days of the week. So you can choose your two days to fast whether they are together or not, let's say Wednesday and Friday. Then, treat all other days as normal days, but on Wednesday and Friday, you eat one or two small meals that together equal 600 calories or less. This is a great beginner diet to try before you get into some more intensive IF. If you're wary of how you may react to fasting, then this method is great to start.

Overview:
- Five days of normal meals according to your daily diet
- Two days of consuming 600 calories or less

The Eat Stop Eat Method

This method was popularized by Brad Pilon and involves a strict 24-hour fast one to two times a week. That is 24 hours of no solid food or caloric intake. Unsweetened coffee and tea are acceptable during the fasting days for this method. A great example would be to fast from dinner to dinner or, let's say, from 4:00 pm to 4:00 pm the next day. It does not matter what time frame you choose, but it should be a solid 24-hour period. Keeping to your usual eating schedule on the non-fasting days is important.

Overview:
- Strict 24-hour fast once or twice a week
- Maintain usual eating schedule during non-fast days

The Alternating Day Method

This method involves fasting every other day. This method can be customized to your liking on the fast days. You can cut back to 600 calories a day, not unlike the 5/2 method, but fasting every other day. If you feel comfortable, you can intake zero calories on the fast days; this would be a very intense method and is not recommended for beginners. For example, eat normally on Sunday, lower calorie intake to 600 calories or less on Monday, eat normally on Tuesday, lower calorie intake Wednesday, eat normally on Thursday, lower calories on Friday. You see, we hit a snag in our pattern as there is an odd number of days in a week. For the odd day out, in this case, Saturday, you can choose to lower the calorie count or eat regularly. It is up to you. For another example, the Saturday odd day out, you could potentially fast for 24 hours then jump back into the pattern on Sunday.

Overview:
- Fast or lower calories every other day
- Keep a usual eating schedule on non-fast days
- Choose what suits you best for the odd day out

The Warrior Method

This method was popularized by Ori Hofmekler. It includes eating small amounts of raw plant-based foods during the day, then one large meal during the evening. Essentially, you are fasting all day and breaking the fast at night. This diet typically focuses on eating raw and unprocessed foods to get the full benefit. For example, during the day, you snack on fruits, veggies, and nuts. Once the evening comes, you prepare a large meal that is as unprocessed and raw as possible.

Overview:
- Light amounts of raw foods or completely fasting during daylight hours
- A large meal at night, as unprocessed and raw as possible

The Spontaneity Method

This method is the loosest and most flexible method of IF. The method is pretty straight forward; there are no guidelines or structures. Simply skip a meal when it's convenient or if you're not hungry. Skipping one or two meals every so often can be a great foundation to lay while you search for a more suitable routine. This method also comes in handy for busy people, parents, or just people who love winging it.

Overview:
- No structure
- Simply skip meals when convenient, or fast whenever you like

Customization Techniques

Now that we have a general idea of different fasting techniques let's keep in mind that these are guidelines that can be customized to fit your specific lifestyle. To reiterate: no one way suits everyone. So as you analyze these methods, keep in mind your personal life and how you alter the structures not only to fit into your schedule but also to personalize your practice. By personalizing your routine, you allow yourself some added empowerment and something that you helped create. Some examples of customizing your practice can include changing the length of fasts, changing diet to suit (vegan, Paleo, etc.), and/or changing the fasting patterns (alternating every two days, etc.).

With the methods above, we see many similarities between them. With the main premise being a caloric restriction and eating window restriction, these methods are simply different customized versions of fasting itself. So this means that we can customize these methods to suit our needs and preferences as individuals.

When we decide to customize a method, it needs to be well thought out. *Why do I need these customizations? Are these customizations feasible as something I can accomplish?* There is an infinite number of ways we can change and alter these techniques, and we will provide some examples below. Keep in mind these are not the only ways to customize but just some basic strategies. Customize as you please, but be safe and mindful in doing so:

- **Customization Strategy #1**: Altering the duration of eating windows

  We see above that one of the main differences in these methods is the timing. For example, the 16/8 method requires eating for eight hours of the day and fasting for sixteen hours of the day. This can be altered easily to suit you. Need a little extra time for the eating window? Add an hour. Feeling confident that you can shorten the eating window? Shorten it an hour or two. You can also choose your eating window during the day. Morning, midday, or night are all suitable times to eat depending on your schedule.

- **Customization Strategy #2**: Altering days

  The days in which you choose to fast are very important but not limited to the guidelines above. The alternating method as an example, alternating days of fasting is a simple pattern, but what if you need two days off from fasting? Make your fast days every third day. Another example would be putting more fast days together, as with the Eat Stop Eat method. Instead of one or two days of complete calorie restriction, maybe do three or push your two days back-to-back for a more challenging fast.

- **Customization Strategy #3**: Altering the timing of meals

Much content online will suggest a proper time for having your meals or will cite the warrior method as an example that requires a large meal at night. This large meal can be placed anywhere in the day according to your preference; in fact, many people prefer their large meal in the middle of the day to avoid a full stomach while sleeping.

- **Customization strategy #4**: Altering meal choices

As noted above, the warrior method requires raw foods to be ingested. Many people have dietary restrictions and preferences that may not fit into these diets and methods, so switch it up! What you eat during your IF routines is important, and you want to keep it healthy. But be reasonable with yourself; choose foods you enjoy. If you prefer fried, greasy foods, maybe try the same ingredients but prepared differently – baked chicken instead of breaded and fried, etc.

- **Customization strategy #5**: Include your lifestyle

When we research fasting online, we see a pattern – health blogs with muscular people in their fitness attire smiling brightly in front of a sunset. This is all fine for some people, but many do not relate to this lifestyle. Lucky for us, fasting is for everyone. You can add fasting to your normal routine easily without hitting the gym or buying spandex. Make it a point to meld IF into your lifestyle rather than view it as something separate from you. Any hobby you love – gaming, fishing, reading, music, art, scrapbooking, etc. – can be a part of your fasting routine. In fact, having a low-intensity hobby is great for the downtime during fasts. Let's not be discouraged if you're not a health nut. Include fasting regardless of your preferred lifestyle, and it will improve it.

These five strategies barely scratch the surface of all the different ways we can alter our routine to fit our lifestyles. Often enough, when we start a fasting routine and get comfortable with the practice, it alters itself naturally to suit our lives. Move with the natural current of things and let your body do the talking. Think deeply on the many strategies available to you and find creative ones to personalize your practice.

We've examined some of the more popular methods of IF and how any method can be altered and customized to fit anyone's needs. While the methods listed above are not the end-all-be-all of IF, they are some of the more popular techniques for a reason. The fitness experts and health gurus that meticulously study and practice these methods present them for the masses online because they work. Another factor being that in our fast-paced society, these methods seem to be some of the better fitting techniques.

Along with promoting these practices, we find much debate online about the validity of fasting and its benefits for the body. Let's explore some common myths and misconceptions.

Chapter 5: Fasting and Exercise Myths Explained

As the popularity of Intermittent Fasting grows, many voices can be heard speaking negatively about the practice. This is understandable as fasting is a taboo in the Western-developed world, seemingly depriving oneself of necessary nutrition would frighten anyone with a conscience. Fears pertaining to exercise are very common. It would seem that not having any food intake would make exercise out of the question, but it will depend on the type of exercise and, of course, your overall health. It is very important to read this section thoroughly, so you don't contradict the work you've done to better yourself. Many myths can be found online, but let's analyze these allegations and apply the science we've learned to debunk any fears and ensure the safest and most effective means of exercise while Intermittent Fasting.

We've seen the science of this kind of fasting allowing our body to use our fat reserves for a cleaner and more efficient energy, but is exercise going to disrupt this process? And if not, what exercises are the most useful? Here we will discuss an IF and exercise combination, while also debunking some other myths pertaining to exercising on an empty stomach.

Let's start with some basic misconceptions about fasting:

Intermittent Fasting Will Slow Your Metabolism

This is a very misunderstood concept. While you fast, your body is going to try to compensate for the disrupted meal routine, but your metabolic rate will not slow; it will simply go about its business as usual. If your body were somehow to use up all its energy and fat reserves, then you would be considered to be 'undereating', and this is when the metabolism slows, and you could be in potential harm's way. So, instead of focusing solely on the idea that fasting is calorie restriction, view it as more of a restriction of the time when you're allowed to intake calories.

By Just Fasting You Will Lose Weight

As we have discussed, losing weight isn't going to happen overnight just because you restrict calories. Developing a nutrient-rich diet alongside casual exercise with IF fasting will be much more effective. Eating pizza every chance you get is not a mindful approach to fasting or a balanced diet, which leads us to the next myth.

You Can Eat Anything You Want In Between Fasts

Ending a fast then diving into a processed food coma is about as counterproductive as it gets. Maintaining healthy eating habits outside of fasting days is going to be a very important key to losing weight and keeping it off. Try to avoid using your fasting practice as an excuse to overindulge.

Intermittent Fasting Is Effective and Everyone Sees Results

This has been a big one throughout the book. No one practice is going to suit everyone. Each individual is very different. Although we all share a basic structure, genes and environment play a huge role in what practices work and what doesn't. Let's not be discouraged though; we can customize our practice and find what works best with just a little time and effort.

Fasting Is Starving Yourself and Unhealthy

We've touched on this one, and it is very common. You express to a peer that you're going to start fasting and they are taken aback by your statement. They think you're going to get hurt or starve to death, and this just isn't true. We've discussed the science, and if used correctly, these ancient practices are safe. Let us keep in mind that we are transforming ourselves through fasting; we are using it as a structure and foundation to a healthy and happy life.

Fasting Leads to Muscle Loss

This is a popular argument for people who oppose fasting. However, the truth is that muscles that are used on a regular basis and plenty of protein ensure the muscle's health. In fact, if the body is searching for fuel, it is not likely to go after muscle since stored fat is way more efficient. Keep in mind, though, that you do not have unlimited fat reserves.

Now, for some myths regarding exercise in general, there is much debate among scientists and people all around the world about what counts as proper exercise and which workouts and regimens are the best. We will continue on our path of 'Everyone is individual and requires customized fitness' as we explore these common misconceptions.

Exercising Leads to Weight Loss

Yes, you need exercise to stay fit, but exercise alone will not suffice. Do not assume that if you eat a pizza, you can simply go 'run it off'. Most studies show that to lose weight, you need balanced eating habits and regular exercise. In fact, many agree that a balanced diet plays an even bigger role in weight loss than the exercise itself.

The Best Time to Exercise Is in the Morning

Exercising in the morning is a popular routine that many people adhere to, but this doesn't mean that it's the best time. Some studies show that exercise in the morning may help prime the body for fat burning during the day, but that's no reason to force a workout in the morning. The best time to exercise is when you feel is the best time. If you like late night runs, go for it. Do what you feel happy doing and make sure to keep active regularly.

Exercise Benefits Only the Physical

Another misconception is that the brain cannot be 'worked out' through exercise. This is untrue. Although puzzles and games help the brain, aerobic exercise seems to be the key to keeping your brain in shape.

Fasted Workouts

With these myths in mind, let's move on to some science about the combination of fasting and exercise or 'fasted workouts'. These workouts are very popular for morning fasts since you can wake up with a relatively empty stomach, have some water, and hit your workout. However, there is much controversy on the subject of exercise on an empty stomach. There are not many studies available on the practice specifically, so the debate continues. Whether or not you think it works better than exercise on a half-full stomach or not, this book is here to give you suitable information to make your own informed decisions.

So, we know that when the stomach is empty, and the body has no immediate access to energy, then it will rely on stored fats. This fact alone implies that working out during a fast would successfully burn unneeded fat reserves, thus leading to weight loss. Although weight loss is the main focus here, we also need to address the many other benefits that IF has when combined with exercise. Studies have shown that fasted cycling to enhance endurance was easier to recover from than endurance cycling with food in the stomach. Along with recovery from endurance exercises, we have seen an improved recovery from the wear and tear of weight training, so we see a pattern of improved recovery after a workout if the athlete was in a fasted state. Similarly, fasted workouts should have higher glycogen storage. By keeping glycogen levels low during workouts, your body adapts to running on low glycogen. Thus, when you have food in your stomach, the body will use its energy more efficiently since it is trained to do so.

These ideas may not be the most amazing practices for a professional athlete, but for a regular person looking to shed a few pounds or develop a new lifestyle, the practices seem optimal.

But what about the many different types of exercise?

Most experts agree that exercise is safe to do while on an empty stomach, but are you getting the most out of your workout? As far as we can tell, the following conclusions can be found:

If your workout requires high levels of speed and power, you will benefit from having food in your stomach. This is due to the high amount of energy you will be burning in a short amount of time, so the energy that is available to be burned quickly is ideal for getting the most out of your workout.

For an empty stomach or fasted workout, the experts suggest cardio and aerobic workouts on all levels, whether it's tai chi or a jog through the park, or intensive yoga and deep stretching. These less intense workouts are ideal practices during a fast and will be the most effective for weight loss.

It is also understood that if you wish to start a fasted cardio routine, you should not have any serious health conditions like low blood pressure or other conditions that may cause dizziness or increase the risk of injury. The following tips are a great guideline for beginners:

    1. Stay hydrated. Consume plenty of water.
    2. Do not work out for longer than an hour
    3. Choose moderate or low-intensity workouts
    4. Listen to your body. If you experience discomfort, then take a breather

In the following chapters, we will reference 'light exercise'. This may be self-explanatory, but it will not hurt to suggest some exercise practices that pair well with IF. These exercises are light and not tough on the body, but we should still break a nice sweat when we are performing these 'light' exercises.

Some fitting ideas for fasted exercise:

- **Yoga**

    Sanskrit for 'union', this traditional Indian practice sets out to unite the body and mind by combining intricate poses and stretches with structured breathing exercises. Cultural influence aside, even spending ten to fifteen minutes a day dedicated to stretching the body and focusing some attention on deep breathing will do wonders as a warmup to a workout or a workout in and of itself.

    You can find plenty of books and online resources to find a yoga practice that suits you. The practice aims to strengthen the body while also furthering flexibility. It is a great core workout and really assists us in getting to know our body and its boundaries.

- **Tai Chi**

As a traditional Chinese martial art, this practice is designed to teach the practitioner how to control and manipulate the subtle energies of the body and its surroundings. Somewhat similar to yoga, this practice involves the constant movement of postures rather than holding poses. Breath is just as important during tai chi as in yoga. As a general rule, being in control of your breathing is a key component to a mindful and healthy life.

There is an abundant amount of material on tai chi online, and many major cities have multiple tai chi instructors and classes that meet in groups or one-on-one. Finding a class that takes place in a natural or relaxing setting is ideal.

- **Jogging**

All of us are familiar with jogging. The casual running exercise aims to build endurance and stamina by running at a steady pace at moderate speeds. Early morning jogs are a great way to start the day and pair well with a fasted morning.

You can jog anywhere. Jog around the block of your neighborhood or visit a school track or a gym that has running space to change the scenery. There are many running groups online if you feel uncomfortable running alone.

- **Cardio**

Cardio workouts are defined as any workout that gets your heart rate up. Jogging can be considered cardio, but there are meticulously designed cardio workouts that aim to burn fat through different intensities. Many workouts ask that you have intervals of intense cardio followed immediately by rest than more intense cardio.

There are hundreds of different cardio styles and workouts available online to suit your skill level and lifestyle. Your local gym should have machines perfect for cardio and possibly even classes dedicated to weight loss through cardio. Cycling machines and the elliptical are popular machines you can find at gyms for cardio workouts.

- **Pilates**

Very similar to yoga, but with more strength building exercises, Pilates was invented in the twentieth century as an effective way to tone muscle without bulking up. It pairs well with IF since it is low impact and can be performed anywhere, not unlike yoga.

Most cities should have Pilates instructors nearby, and there are abundant resources online.

- **Hiking**

This is a low-impact, relaxing, and thought-provoking activity. Taking a hike in the woods is an immersive experience. There's something very beneficial about being in a natural setting away from all the hustle and bustle of a town or city. Depending on the terrain, hiking can be a casual stroll or close to a treacherous climb. The combination of fasting and hiking is an amazing one as you notice your senses are heightened as you walk empty-bellied through the forest.

There are hiking trails all around the world, and they often state the intensity level of the hike. Searching for new trails and scenic spots quickly becomes a hobby that is beneficial on many levels. Adventurous, educational, self-reflective, and most certainly great for your body, hiking is paired wonderfully with IF since you are in control of how difficult it is. But, of course, if you are fasting and going out into the woods, be sure to bring plenty of water and emergency snacks.

Chapter 6: Best Foods for Fasting

Moving forward, as we get ever closer to our goal of completely changing our outlook on the diet, we find ourselves with a bit of an appetite. But what foods are okay to eat while fasting? Although you could safely keep your normal diet and simply fast around it, we can optimize our transformation by including foods that are ideal to pair with a diet that includes regular Intermittent Fasting. With access to nearly any food we desire, it is tough not to grab the pizza slice or burger when we feel hungry. However, we're developing our confidence and control here, not simply fulfilling our immediate desires. By taking control of our instant desires, we empower ourselves to think mindfully of our next meal, and a dedicated IF regime assists us in accomplishing this life-altering goal.

First things first, let's take a moment to think about our diets. Go back one week and write out all the meals you had including snacks and contemplate it:

Were these foods I desired? Were these foods of convenience? Were there any foods that could have been easily left out? Were these foods rich in nutrients?

These questions are pretty straightforward, but let's try and be more abstract:

Where did the food come from? Was this food natural? What time of the day was I eating? Was it a set routine? Why did I choose these particular foods? Was this the same diet I've maintained for over a decade?

This contemplation should be thorough and invigorating. There will be realizations and even more questions, more intimate ones. Let the thought process flow over you. This is a beginning step to being mindful of your diet. These simple questions will help prepare you for how your diet will change once IF begins. You will consciously change your habits, but you will also subconsciously be building a relationship with your desires and changing them from the inside out. Keep your diet in mind leading up to the fast and consider some options below if they haven't been in your diet before.

Many fad diets come and go over the years, but in reality, they are just that – fads. Cutting out carbs or only eating protein isn't going to give us the well-rounded, transformative effect we're searching for here. We need to balance our diet, explore nutrient-rich ingredients, and find alternatives to the ingredients that are most detrimental to our goals.

Moving forward, let us investigate what type of diets are best suited for IF. Since it requires you only to eat during certain parts of the day or only on certain days, we need not to just stuff ourselves with whatever we get our hands on but to be mindful of how balanced our meals are. Since we aim to lose weight while simultaneously transforming the way we view meals and food, we need meals and snacks that are mostly unprocessed, high in fiber, and have lean protein. But what we eat isn't the only factor. If you think about a 'normal' day of eating, you will realize that our digestive system is working from morning until night to digest three or more meals a day. This is just asking for weight gain since our stomachs are never empty, and our body doesn't need to burn our fat reserves for energy. So, we soon realize that the time we eat is also important. The timing will be covered in subsequent chapters.

As we think about raw, nutrient-rich food, we also consider where our food comes from. Foods produced locally will be richer in nutrients and promote the local economy by supporting smaller farms. This is a practice in mindfulness as we seek to develop a better relationship with food and, through this mindful notion, contribute to a more ecologically and economically balanced world around us. Since we seek to better ourselves through transformation, our relationship with food needs to be reevaluated, and an excellent place to start is where your food is sourced. You will also learn more about the foods available to you, educating yourself on which foods are in the season, thus helping you decide what foods you will be preparing during fasting weeks. Taking a visit to your local farmer's market is more than likely the best option for sourcing local foods, not to mention the relationship you build with other people who share the same notion of community support.

Here are some foods that are rich in nutrients and are ideal for a fasting lifestyle:

Leafy Greens

Deep, dark, leafy greens are a staple in the optimized fasting diet. These foods are rich in vitamins A, C, and K as well as plenty of potassium and fiber. These greens can replace the standard lettuce in any recipe and are available all year round. Kale, among many other leafy greens, is even considered one of the most nutrient-rich foods known to humans. If you are not a fan of the flavor of leafy greens, blend them up in a smoothie with some fruits to mask the taste.

Some examples of delicious leafy greens include kale, spinach, collard greens, chard, turnip greens, and cabbage.

Garlic

Garlic is found in many recipes and can be eaten raw if you don't mind the pungent flavor and aroma. High in B vitamins, vitamin C, calcium, copper, and selenium, this nutrient-rich food could potentially lower and balance blood pressure while also containing antibacterial and antifungal properties. Garlic can be a welcome ingredient in most meals, minced or whole.

Potatoes

Potatoes are versatile and fun to cook with. They pack a massive amount of potassium, copper, and iron while also containing a good amount of vitamins B and C. Another ideal factor for IF is how filling a potato can be. Try boiling potatoes for the most beneficial preparation method.

Tomatoes

With a wide variety of different types to choose from, tomatoes are versatile and yield many different flavors. Packed full of vitamins and minerals, these beautifully bright foods can be eaten raw by themselves or added to salads.

Broccoli

Notorious for being hated by many people, broccoli is full of vitamins C and K among other vitamins and minerals. Best steamed or eaten raw in salads.

Cauliflower

Cauliflower is an incredibly nutrient-rich food that deserves way more attention. Vitamin C, K, B12, and filled with fiber, this vegetable has much-needed minerals and small amounts of protein. Find creative recipes online or eat raw in salads.

Sunflower Seeds

An excellent source of vitamin E, these tiny seeds are great to snack on. Antioxidants, copper, phosphorous, and magnesium abound in these little seeds. Add to any salad or eat raw.

Almonds

Nuts and seeds are wonderful for snacking during IF. Almonds, in particular, pack a bunch of vitamin E, copper, magnesium, and fiber. One downside is the large number of calories, so be cautious while on a restricted caloric intake and snacking on almonds.

Blueberries

Among the many berries and their many benefits, blueberries stand out when it comes to being rich in nutrients. Although not as rich in vitamins as most vegetables, blueberries boast a wild amount of antioxidants, which can protect the brain and repair cells. Throw some blueberries in a salad or snack on them raw.

Raspberries

Although a little tough to find in some places, if you can get your hands on some raspberries, you can fulfill your body's needs for vitamin C, fiber, and manganese. Eat raw, with yogurt, or in smoothies.

Chocolate

You're probably thinking of name brands of candy bars right now, but in all seriousness, dark chocolate is packed with antioxidants, fiber, iron, magnesium, and copper. Grabbing chocolate with 80% or higher cocoa content is the healthiest. Mix it with smoothies, nuts, or eat raw.

Beans

Beans, black beans, in particular, are filled with iron and protein. They are filling and great to replace red meats for protein content that is much leaner. Plenty of minerals and folic acid come along with the versatile bean. Cook in chili, burritos, or even salads.

Rice

Among other whole grains, rice is rich in fiber and small amounts of vitamins and minerals. Rice is one of the most consumed foods in the world and can be mixed and paired with almost anything. Sweet or savory, rice goes a long way when fasting. It is filling, inexpensive, and easy to cook. Pair with sautéed vegetables, fish, tofu, and beans.

Tofu

Fermented soybean doesn't sound appealing to everyone, but tofu is incredibly versatile and is a great source of lean, plant-based protein. As a great alternative to red meats and other animal proteins, tofu is a lynchpin in a vegetarian or vegan diet. Marinate and sauté with veggies or press and fry for sandwiches.

Salmon

Salmon stands out among fish as a nutrient-rich powerhouse. Filled with omega-3 fatty acids and plenty of protein, salmon also helps lower heart disease. Replace beef or other meats with salmon two to three times a week for a leaner, more nutrient-rich protein source.

Shellfish

Shellfish may be the most nutritious sea creatures we know of. Clams, oysters, and mussels, among others, rank high on the oceanic food list. Excellent sources of B12 and other vitamins, these foods also contain a ton of zinc, potassium, and iron. Consume sparingly perhaps on a celebratory night out or during other special occasions.

The foods mentioned above are some of the highest valued foods for IF. Work them into your diet as well as you can, and don't be afraid to get creative with preparation techniques. Keep note of the foods that you already have in your diet and the ones you want to add to your new diet.

Meal Prepping

Along with developing a balanced and fast-friendly diet, there are techniques to take the complicated process of preparing and cooking every meal. Meal prepping, or simply meal prep, is an excellent way to save time during busy weeks, especially if you are implementing your new IF regimen. This technique is pretty straightforward: prepare all your meals for a week and store them in a container until they are ready to use. As simple as this is, let's go over some steps that often get overlooked to get you started. We will keep this step-by-step list focused on IF for the sake of our goals.

Step #1: Decide what food you want to prep

Make a list of mostly raw or unprocessed foods that you wish to consume throughout the upcoming week. Are you having the same meal every day? Or are you switching it up day to day? Once you decide what you wish to prep, head to the grocery store and be sure to buy plenty for a week's worth of meals. Some people like to choose a calorie limit and choose meals that stay under a certain caloric intake per meal. Once you have the meals in mind, continue on.

Step#2: Choose a day to prep

Your refrigerator is stocked, and you're ready to prep. Find out when your fast begins and prepare the food the day before you start. This way, the food will stay fresh longer into your week-long fast.

Step#3: Obtain containers

You will need containers to keep your prepared meals in. Tupperware and the other storage ware you have available will suffice, but many buy containers that have divided sections for the different foods. The containers need to be airtight and BPA-free. Here's a short list of features your containers should have:

- BPA-free
- Reusable
- Microwave safe
- Stackable

Once you have your containers, you can start preparing the food.

Step#4: Prepare food

It's the day before you start your fast, so take your chosen ingredients and prepare them as you wish. Divide the foods out in seven equal parts for each day of the week, and then put them in the containers and store in the refrigerator. Keep in mind that uncooked foods will keep fresh longer and also pick things that will not require any further cooking or preparation once it's time to eat. Of course, having to reheat sometimes is necessary.

Step#5: Begin your week

You have your meals ready to go, and you don't need to worry about what to eat for a whole seven days. It's a nice relief – just don't forget to bring your prepared meal with you if you leave the house!

Meal prepping is a great way to keep control of your calorie intake and organize a new IF routine. With such a structured technique, it's nearly impossible to slip up on your goals. The steps above are a great foundation for an

IF week. Alter the steps and quantities as you need to according to your fasting guidelines.

Below we will recommend some foods that are perfect for meal prep. Let's discuss the main courses and recommend some suitable examples of ingredients for these times of the day. The reference guide below will be focused on mostly raw unprocessed foods.

Breakfast

Breakfast is thought to be the most important meal of the day. However, this idea is flawed because it takes an entire balanced day of food to create a healthful life. No one meal is any important than the other; they all work together to create health and fulfillment. For our purposes in this book, we want breakfast foods that will not bog us down, so avoiding meats, bread, and sugary foods is ideal. With these things in mind let's take a look at some nutrient-rich foods that are great for starting the day:

- **Fruits:** Yes, we're avoiding sweets, but the natural source of sugar in fruit is a world away from the refined sugars we find in breakfast cereals and processed milk. An apple on the go is simple and quick. Cutting some orange slices or melon the night before is a great way to have a quick bite in the morning. Fruits are fulfilling and bursting with flavor, so for an IF regimen they come in handy as a quick source of energy or a light snack for an empty stomach.

    To be clear, we are talking about raw fruits – not jellies or preserves, not an Apple Danish. Having fruit chopped and ready to eat in the refrigerator is a great habit to get into. A huge bowl of fruit salad is exceptionally tantalizing after a long fasting day.

    Preparation: raw, fruit salad, paired with peanut butter, smoothie

Acceptable fruits: apples, watermelon, honeydew, cantaloupe, oranges, clementine, cherries, bananas (although bananas have the most sugar content)

- **Berries:** There are plenty of common misconceptions and confusion about whether or not berries are fruits. They technically are, but we'll give them a special section all to themselves. The protocol for berries is the same as fruit: have them raw or mixed in a salad.

Preparation: raw, dried, salad, paired with other fruits, smoothie

Acceptable berries: blackberry, strawberry, blueberry

- **Nuts and Seeds:** Like fruits, nuts and seeds make for a quick raw snack that can easily be taken on the go. When choosing nuts, be sure to pick ones that are not covered with sugar or flavors. So avoid chocolate-covered or honey-roasted versions. Sea-salted nuts and raw nuts are the best.

Preparation: raw or roasted, trail mix, paired with fruits, smoothie

Nutritious nuts: almonds, cashews, pistachios, pecans, pumpkin seeds, sunflower seeds, chia seed, hemp seed

- **Whole Grains:** There are many whole grains to choose from, and these grains offer a lot in the way of fiber and carious vitamins. It is wise to eat bread sparingly, but a nice whole grain slice will go a long way; perhaps even switch bread out for a lighter option like a tortilla. The versatility of rice is a lifesaver if you're on a budget.

Preparation: cooked into oatmeal, bread, rice dishes, paired with almost anything.

Nutritious whole grains: rice, corn, oats, quinoa

- **Water:** This is an obvious ingredient, but also just as the only thing you have in the morning, water is a great way to start the day. Just a couple of 8-oz glasses and you're good to go – no harm in skipping out on breakfast every once in a while.

- **Eggs:** With eggs in the morning, we're getting to some heavier, less ideal breakfast foods. For a leaner egg, avoid eating the yolk. But if you must have eggs and need something a little bit heavier, eggs offer a high-protein inexpensive kick-start to the day.

    Preparation: soft boiled, egg white omelet with veggies

- **Honorable Mention – Black Coffee:** Although it's a surprise, coffee is actually very healthy for you, not to mention an awesome way to start the day with its complex flavors and caffeine content. Of course, for our purposes, we will not be adding sugar, syrups, or milk to our coffee. It is highly recommended to develop a palette for black coffee and buy yourself a coffee as organic and locally roasted as possible.

Breakfast is simple. It is not necessary to eat steak, eggs, and potatoes for breakfast to 'start your day right'. Give the body some time to ease into the day by staying light and rich in nutrients for your breakfast choices.

Lunch

Midday meals are important to those who work long days and need a much-needed break. This leads to many of us settling for fast foods and sandwiches that have little nutritional value. For those who are fasting much of the time, the first solid food intake of the day is during lunchtime, so the choices we make for this meal will influence greatly how our day turns out. Meal prepping and smoothies can save you from settling for less healthy and processed foods.

- **Fruits and Berries:** These two food groups are going to show up a lot, so let's get used to it. These sweet foods are great for those with a nagging sweet tooth, not to mention a great source of quick energy.

Preparation: raw, dried, salad, paired with other fruits, smoothie

Acceptable berries: blackberry, strawberry, blueberry

- **Vegetables:** With such a wide variety to choose from, there is a veggie for everyone. Rich in fiber and various vitamins, vegetables are an IF's best friend. We can chat all day about the variety of ways vegetables can be prepared and consumed, but for a midday meal, salad is King.

Preparation: steamed or sautéed, eaten raw or with salad

Nutritious vegetables: tomatoes, broccoli, Brussel sprouts, potatoes, kale, carrots, spinach, cauliflower

- **Nuts and Seeds:** Like fruits, nuts and seeds make for a quick raw snack that can easily be taken on the go. When choosing nuts, be sure to pick ones that are not covered with sugar or flavors. So avoid chocolate-covered or honey-roasted versions. Sea-salted nuts and raw nuts are the best.

Preparation: raw or roasted, trail mix, paired with fruits, smoothie

Nutritious nuts: almonds, cashews, pistachios, pecans, pumpkin seeds, sunflower Seeds, chia seed, hemp seed

- **Whole Grains:** There are many different whole grains to choose from, and these grains offer a lot in the way of fiber and carious vitamins. It is wise to eat breads sparingly, but a nice whole grain slice will go a long way perhaps even switch bread out for a lighter option like a tortilla. The versatility of rice is a lifesaver if you're on a budget.

Preparation: cooked into oatmeal, bread, rice dishes, paired with almost anything.

Nutritious whole grains: rice, corn, oats, quinoa

- **Chicken:** Very lean and readily available, chicken is carbohydrate free and has very little fat and calorie content. It is an easy transition to cut out red meats and replace them with chicken. It's easy to prepare and versatile.

Preparation: boiled, sautéed, not breaded, tossed in a salad

Nutritious chicken: Not breaded, lightly seasoned, free range

Dinner

The last full meal of the day, dinner/supper is typically reserved for heavy meals and entertaining guests. The evening meal sets the tone of the evening and often is the meal that is most well thought out throughout the day. Steaks, burgers, and other heavy entrées rule this meal in the Western world, but we want to find leaner and more nutritious options for our purposes.

- **Fish:** Eating fish in place of heavier, less lean meats is a great way to alter your evening diet for the fasting lifestyle. In place of steaks, burgers, and pork, substitute the more nutrient-rich and lighter variety of fish or seafood.

  Nutritious fish: salmon, albacore, sardines, trout, oysters

  Preparation: Cooked thoroughly, sautéed or steam
- **Chicken:** Very lean, and readily available, chicken is carbohydrate free and has very little fat and calorie content. It is an easy transition to cut out red meats and replace them with chicken. It's easy to prepare and versatile.

  Preparation: boiled, sautéed, not breaded

  Nutritious chicken: not breaded, lightly seasoned, free range
- **Tofu:** The go-to replacement for meat-based protein, tofu is a soybean product that is full of great protein. It is a staple in Eastern cultures, and the Western world is slowly getting on board. Tofu is almost flavorless by itself, but when marinated or combined with veggies in a rice dish, it's just as valuable as any meat.
- **Vegetables:** With such a wide variety to choose from, there is a veggie for everyone. Rich in fiber and various vitamins,

vegetables are an IF's best friend. We can chat all day about the variety of ways vegetables can be prepared and consumed, but for an evening meal, a salad appetizer or a sautéed side dish are winners.

Preparation: steamed or sautéed

Nutritious vegetables: tomatoes, broccoli, Brussel sprouts, potatoes, kale, carrots, spinach, cauliflower

- **Whole Grains:** There are many different whole grains to choose from, and these grains offer a lot in the way of fiber and carious vitamins. It is wise to eat breads sparingly, but a nice whole grain slice will go a long way, perhaps even switch bread out for a lighter option like a tortilla. The versatility of rice is a lifesaver if you're on a budget.

Preparation: cooked into oatmeal, bread, rice dishes, paired with almost anything

Nutritious whole grains: rice, corn, oats, quinoa

This basic guide to what foods are best at which part of the day is great for developing your own diet plan.

Snacks

Light snacks throughout the day help to appease your appetite and offer a much-needed break from monotonous days. Keeping snack foods handy is also a practice and also for safety – just in case your fasting days get the best of you, and you find yourself losing all your energy. Although it's popular to keep processed snacks nearby, chips, candies, and sodas are not ideal or our goals at hand.

Preparation: raw, trail mix, organic prepackaged

Nutritious snacks: nuts, seeds, fruits, veggies, granola, dark chocolate

Notable Diets

With weight loss in mind, we should explore some popular diets that pair quite well with IF. There are a few diets that have hit the mainstream and come equipped with the guidelines and structure needed to optimize weight loss when paired with IF. While diets have served as the stand-in for what it takes to be healthy in recent decades, studies have shown that simply altering what foods you eat will not lead to a healthful and balanced life. Many subtle changes need to be implemented to achieve these goals. Yes, the food you eat is very important, but it's not the end-all-be-all of healthful practices. Going on a diet for a month doesn't change your life. If you want a healthy life and wish to maintain that health, you will need to balance all aspects of health – not just the food you eat. Below we will explore some diets and how they are perfect for IF.

Mediterranean Diet

This diet is inspired by the foods and nutritional outlook of people living near the Mediterranean Sea. Fruits, legumes, vegetables, and other plant-based foods rule this diet, along with an abundant amount of extra-virgin olive oil and fresh fish.

As it is well known, the culture and societies surrounding the Mediterranean are joyous about their meals, not to mention red wines. The celebratory nature of their lifestyles is no doubt key in their health and happiness. This mindful attitude is exactly what we aim for when it comes to our own relationships with food. The positive mindset, vegetables, fresh lean protein, and plenty of healthy fats make this diet, as well as the cultures that influence it, ideal for IF.

Paleo Diet

The Paleo diet, or caveman diet, is one of the more popular diets that has seen its fifteen minutes of fame but has continued onward after its initial boom in the mainstream media. The diet is loosely based on what we think our ancient ancestors consumed before agriculture and farming was developed. As far as studies go, it is thought that our ancestors were extremely active and ate a diet of organic and wild meats, nuts, greens, and even insects.

Many assume that the prehistoric man thrived mainly on meat, but this is a common misconception. Hunting alone would not yield enough food for a large tribe, so it's commonly thought that less than half of the diet would consist of meat. The rest of the diet would be filled with foraged foods like plants, berries, seeds, and nuts. Considering different regions around the world and the vague nature of studying the past, there is a lot of difference in opinion when it comes to the Paleo diet. It is safe to say that not all hunts would be successful, so there would be prolonged instances of sustaining on nothing but plant-based foods. This pattern of eating, in essence, is IF. So the Paleo diet has a history with IF, but how can we apply this to the modern world?

There is no one strict structure for the Paleo diet. And given the variety of diets in the ancient world, on a scale from low-carb, high animal content to high-carb plant-based, many different styles can be considered 'paleo'. So, here is a general outline for what foods to eat with a basic Paleo diet:

- Meat (fish, lamb, beef, chicken, seafood)
- Eggs (free range, cage free)
- Vegetables (potatoes, broccoli, carrots, tomatoes)
- Nuts and Seeds (almonds, walnuts, sunflower seeds, pumpkin seeds)
- Fruits (apples, pears, oranges, avocados)
- Healthy Oils (extra virgin olive oil, coconut oil)
- Herbs (sea salt, rosemary, turmeric, garlic)

This list is a great stepping stone to more specific guidelines, and keep in mind this food should be as organic as possible, and the fruits, nuts, and herbs being wild foraged, of course. For a stricter regimen, here is a list of foods to avoid:

- Legumes (beans, lentils, peanuts)
- Grains (bread, pasta, wheat, rye, barley)
- Dairy (some diets allow butter and cheese)

- Some oils (soybean, corn, sunflower, grapeseed)
- Artificial sweeteners (sucralose, aspartame)
- Very processed foods (frozen, prepackaged, additives)

Ketogenic Diets

As we discussed briefly, ketosis is when your body has used up all its quick energy and creates ketones to help burn stored fat. Typically, these diets are all about high-fat, low-carbohydrate meals, like plenty of eggs, avocados, and fatty meats, while avoiding bread and whole grains which are the prime source of carbs in the contemporary diet.

By cutting back our carbohydrate consumption to 60 grams or less per day for four to five days, our body will begin to produce ketones, which allow the body to use stored fat. The body cannot directly use the fat on its own. This diet, paired with an IF routine, can be very effective for our weight loss purposes. However, we need to take into account the dangers that ketosis can be present for certain people. Avoid inducing ketosis if you have diabetes, are taking high blood pressure medication, or breastfeeding.

Vegetarian Diets

Vegetarian diets are popular all around the world and in many countries and cultures. Even within the scope of the Paleo diet, vegetarianism is acceptable at times. The diet is not only a healthy alternative to contemporary Western diets but is also more ecologically friendly compared to a diet where all the protein comes from animal-based sources. Many vegetarians choose this diet for the health benefits and their overall wellbeing, but many people find themselves practicing this diet for their love of animals and the earth.

As you are more than likely aware, the vegetarian's diet has a strict no-meat rule. This means no beef, pork, fish, chicken, or any other meat. Many vegetarians still consume eggs, eat butter, and use milk, but strictly no meat itself is consumed. Much of the scientific motivation behind the vegetarian diet is that plant-based proteins are better for you and easier to digest than red meats. Although this diet is just as balanced as any other, when approaching a vegetarian diet, it is important that you eat plenty of protein to make up for the immense amount of protein lost when cutting out meats. Another issue is iron and sodium intake that is found abundantly in meat. These building blocks of life need extra attention with a vegetarian diet. Regardless of motivation, the vegetarian diet is great for IF, with all the nutrient-rich ingredients found in the world of animal-free sustenance.

Vegan Diet

Another animal-free diet, the vegan diet is similar to the vegetarian diet, but instead of simply cutting out meat itself, this diet requires that you cut out all animal products. Eggs, milk, butter, and anything with the slightest bit of animal-related ingredients are off limits. This an extreme version of vegetarianism and even crosses over into other territories besides the individual's diet. Many vegans take pride in their decision to avoid all animal products every moment of their lives – no fur clothing, no products tested on animals, absolutely nothing that uses animals. This diet comes with a philosophy, and here in this book, our goals are elsewhere. There is plenty of information online about veganism.

The Whole30 Diet

This diet has seen a surge in popularity in recent years with the 'gluten-free' trend that has been going around. The diet itself calls for us to eliminate foods that are common culprits when it comes to allergies and intolerances. So it means cutting out gluten-rich grains and legumes like beans and peanuts. The diet involves a 30-day 'clean eating' cycle where you cut these potentially unhealthy foods out of your diet for 30 days, then see how you feel. You can gradually reintroduce these foods and again take note of your body's reactions. This diet can almost allow us to see if we are intolerant to certain foods, thus allowing us to cut out troublesome ingredients. This is also a great diet for developing mindfulness and awareness about our bodies. It will pair well with an IF week at the end of the 30-day cycle.

Raw Food Diet

The raw food diet is very similar to the vegan diet, and many vegans adhere to its basic principle of eating foods in their natural form. It includes raw fruits, vegetables, nuts, and seeds. Uncooked and not dehydrated or seasoned, the nutritional value of these foods in this diet cannot be debated. This diet is a pretty simple one, but it is more than likely a world away from your current diet. Some may find it difficult not to cook, and without cooking your meal choices are limited. This diet will be one of the more difficult to uphold, not to mention one of the more difficult diets to practice and also ensure that you get all the needed nutrients. However, if you feel like the raw food diet suits you, try it out and pay very close attention to what your body says in return.

With the incredible variety of diets available online, there's no shortage of plans, routines, and fads. It is best to avoid choosing a diet based on popularity and choose diets that you will actually enjoy. There's no reason to take all the joy out of eating and the art of cooking in exchange for a routine that may not even be very effective. With this in mind, we can safely say that if you find that a diet needs a little customization to suit your needs, then go ahead and alter it. This is your practice; this is your life. Take control and empower yourself regardless of what people say. Enjoyment of food and your lifestyle choices are just as important as the choices themselves. If we are not taking pleasure out of our choices, then we need to rearrange and alter our current routine.

Once we have established our preferred dietary choices or altered our diet to one with foods that are more suitable for IF, we can begin making preparations to start our fasting week.

Chapter 7: Getting Started

So, we've made it. We stand now with enough valuable information and proper preparation for setting a date to start including Intermittent Fasting in our daily lives. This does not mean we have to fast every day, but fasting is on our mind and a part of our lives. By spending a little time out of the day to be mindful and contemplate our relationship with IF, we further our confidence and can develop a firm grasp of our goals and aspirations. Not only is maintaining awareness of our body and mind important to our goals in this book, but also an important practice to implement every day. Our mindset and perception of a situation affect us subtly.

We emphasize awareness and mindfulness so much in this book for a good reason. We see the ancient cultures using fasting to great success, and it is certain that their practices in mindfulness and awareness are key to this success. Old practices like meditation and deep thought were very important to overall wellbeing in ancient philosophy. And so, as we see our ancestors and their practices permeating our current world, being studied in scientific settings and utilized in everyday life, we must give credit where credit is due and acknowledge that these practices are a very important aspect of existence. While keeping this in mind, let's move forward. Here, we begin the physical journey. We need to choose what type of fast works for us, schedule our meals, and then begin.

First things first, how do you want to fast? Choosing a practice type will be tough, at first, and more often than not, the first course of action is not the one we stick with. Depending on work, family, and other important influences, we can choose one of the styles in the previous chapter and work with it and see it change as we do. You can do a little customization there, some slight changes here. It is your practice, so do what you feel is best for you and not what everyone else is doing. We cannot tell you everything to do, but here are some helpful tips for the weeks leading up to the first fast:

> 1. **Think about it.** Think of yourself and what you want to accomplish. Consider your consumption and how it affects your body and mind. Prepare mentally for challenges that you will face – hunger, physical changes, emotions, and other drastic changes – that accompany this practice.
> 2. **Prepare physically.** If you find that you're are in poor health, you may want to start changing little things in the week or two leading up to the fast. Cut back on desserts and detrimental foods, take a walk and other casual exercises, or chat with friends and family about what you're trying to accomplish to find support.
> 3. **Meal prep.** Many people find that organizing meals beforehand helps keep them on track. Buying reusable containers and preparing a week's worth of meals to keep in the fridge helps save time and ensures you keep your diet right for the fast.
> 4. **Ease in.** Many feel that jumping right into a fast is shocking to their bodies, so the week before your major fast, maybe do half of what you planned for the big week. Maybe pick a fasting technique and use it for one or two days.

By preparing yourself beforehand, there's less of a chance that you will fail or have to restart the fast. You will be ready for any changes or unexpected outcomes that may find their way to you. Do not be disheartened if you cannot complete a fast the first time around. Everyone is different, and some people take the calorie restriction easier than others. If you have issues getting started, do not give up. Change your plan as you see fit, even if you only make it twenty-five percent of the week, you still have begun your transformation; you have still started changing your life for the better. The subtlest of changes have begun as soon as you started thinking about changing yourself. Be confident in yourself and your convictions. It's quite all right to fail; this is where we learn the most about ourselves. In fact, failing can even be viewed as an exercise in mindfulness. You learn from your mistakes and can try a different approach the next time around. All in all, do not give up. If you truly value yourself and your life, then this should be plenty of motivation to continue onward until you have reached your goals. Having prepared yourself mentally and physically, success is inevitable.

Once we have given our schedule, lifestyle, and personal needs some thorough thought, we need to think even deeper about our personal goals. Are you seeking simply to lose a few pounds? Are you only curious about IF and not sure about the beginning? How will starting a fasting routine affect your lifestyle and the people around you? The questions are infinite in this context, but for all our intents and purposes with this book, we have a loose set of goals that we aim to achieve:

- Ridding ourselves of excess fat
- Developing a mindful and aware perception of health
- Adjusting our diets to suit a healthful lifestyle
- Maintaining any progress we achieve (keep weight off, maintain awareness)
- Through the combination of the goals above transform our lives for the better

This list is presented as a general and vague overview of our intentions with this book. Even if you really only want to lose a few pounds, doing so will also transform your mindset and awareness, whether it's intentional or not. Develop a personal list with the above goals in mind. The list can be anything you want to change: weight loss, health, new job, new home, etc. Anything you desire, add it to this list and think about how a healthier lifestyle can affect these things. From the mundane to the most important, feel free to be as specific as you need to be with your goals. You can apply these lifestyle changes to other aspects of your life too. Improving your health is inevitably going to touch all corners of your life, so setting goals outside the scope of physical health is quite all right. As we move forward let's also take time to visualize ourselves as the people we wish to be. Visualize yourself at peak performance, visualize your life and surroundings as you truly want to be. This image will act as motivation and also as a primer for your mindfulness practice. The body and mind work together as one, so treat them as equals as we embark on our newfound Intermittent Fasting lifestyle.

Now that we have a solid idea of what we aim to achieve, we can begin taking action to start our IF routine. The guide below will take all the methods we've explored and lay out weeklong step-by-step instructions for each method.

Chapter 8: One Week Step-by-Step Guide

Now that we've gotten started and prepared our minds and bodies let's take a look at a step-by-step guide covering seven days of Intermittent Fasting. Here, we will provide a seven-day guide for each of the methods mentioned in the previous chapter. We will start the guides out with a 'preparation day', being the day before the first day of your fasting week. This day allows us to ground ourselves and prepare physically and mentally for the week to come. This guide can act as a quick reference guide during your journey, as well as a strict guideline for the various types of Intermittent Fasting.

Accompanying these guides will be some suggestions for customizing your practice. Customization techniques also come in handy to personalize your routine. A thoughtful approach to this would be to make your practice distinct and in tune with your wishes and goals. We will explore some customization techniques below, but feel free to be creative and use your best judgment. Do your research, listen to your body, and, as always, be mindful.

With the following guide, we will suggest good times for exercise according to the information we have learned over the course of this book. Let's keep in mind that this is simply a guide and does not particularly have to be followed strictly. Any suggestions for meal timing, non-caloric drinks, or exercise are only loose guidelines based on the science and studies we have analyzed. Being aware that not everyone has the same schedule, we will do our best to make the guide concise and easy to fit into your daily routine. Be creative with customization and always have plenty of water available!

The following lists will give seven-day examples for a few of the Intermittent Fasting methods mentioned above.

The 16/8 Method

Guideline:

- Fast sixteen hours per day
- Eating window eight hours per day
- Non-caloric drinks acceptable
- Stay hydrated
- Exercise first thing in the morning

With the 16/8 method, you will be fasting for around sixteen hours out of the 24-hour day, which leaves an eating window of around eight hours. Obviously, your fasting hours will include the amount of time that you sleep. We will focus on one popular arrangement of this method where your eight-hour eating window is in the evening. This is probably the easiest way to go about this method, especially if combined with exercise in the morning.

Sunday

For our guide here, you will start with Sunday. Although you are not fasting on this day, you still want to prepare yourself for the upcoming week. Be sure to remember what time your last meal is today. Sixteen hours from that time, you will begin your eating window. Have your schedule for tomorrow mentally prepared or written down. Although exercise isn't mandatory, we have discussed the added benefits of physical activity, and, for our main goal of weight loss, we will include exercise for this guide. We also would like to suggest eating light, easily digestible foods on this day for this will help you better adapt to the upcoming week. For our purposes here, let's say you finished your last meal at seven PM. This gives you until eleven AM at the earliest to have a bite to eat. You can see how this arrangement is very fitting for standard nine-to-five jobs.

Key Points:

- Remember or take note of the time of your last meal.
- Eat light, easily digestible foods on this day.
- Keep notes on the progress.

Monday (Day 1)

Morning. Upon waking up, start your day with a glass or two of water to your liking. If coffee or tea is an important part of your morning, it is fine to have as long as there is no sugar or milk added. The morning is a perfect time to exercise, the stomach is empty, and the remaining quick energy sources from any previous meals will be easily burned off, and we can start burning fat reserves. Most people will likely have to work during the week, so be sure to have access to plenty of water. We will note here that if your work requires a large amount of energy and power, this method may not be the most suitable.

Midday. If this is your first fast, you will surely be feeling the effects. Those circadian rhythms we were discussing are realizing that this is not a normal day and will adapt accordingly. Although you may feel strange, keep in mind that this is a transformative experience and will not go without some strange or unknown feelings. Noon is coming around, so we're well into our eating window. We officially have until seven PM to eat a few meals. So, have a standard lunch you would typically consume or even upgrade to a more fast-friendly meal with the suggestions for foods above. Notice the taste of your meal and really engage with the food on an intimate level. Does it feel different as you eat? Are flavors more or less intense? Keep note of any changes in perception or feeling. After lunch, feel free to snack as you please – it's your eating window!

Evening. As the evening approaches, you can continue to snack or have meals, but most people feel comfortable having two to three meals during this time; you can adjust this to your liking. Once seven PM comes around, be sure to wind down and cease to intake any calories for the next sixteen hours.

Key Points:

- Be mindful of your body and the start of your new routine.
- Keep mental or physical notes on your experiences and changes in general.
- Stay hydrated.
- Remember the times of last caloric intake.

Tuesday (Day 2)

Morning. Upon awakening, you may repeat the previous day's routine – non-caloric drinks, exercise – but no eating until eleven AM. This morning will be very similar to Monday as we are just now starting to get into the fast. Today may be less intense as far as your body goes as it is adjusting naturally to the new IF routine. Keep notes on your morning experiences. Is it easier or more difficult to get out of bed in the morning? Are you more energetic or do you feel drained? If you have an exercise routine, is it easier or more difficult? How do you feel after the workout? Being aware of the changes you feel is important during the fasting experience. Any negative feelings or discomfort should be noted as well as positive experiences.

Midday. Your eating window approaches just in time for the standard lunchtime. As with the previous day, keep an open mind and be aware of your experiences. Again, stick with meals that you would typically eat or upgrade your meals to more nutrient-rich foods.

Evening. The second evening is here, and you're still within your eating window. Be aware of the many changes and be sure to keep up with the current pattern and be relatively strict with the routine you have.

Key Points:
- Be mindful and take notes on your feelings.
- Keep up with your routine and time patterns.
- Stay hydrated.

Wednesday (Day 3)

Morning. The third morning commences, and the routine is becoming a part of your normal routine. With all the intense writing online about the dangers of IF, we approach the third morning noticing that this transformative practice is really not that difficult but simply requires a little attention to detail and self-discipline. Live the morning as you do, go about the day as usual, and pay attention to any changes or feelings that are notable.

Midday. Lunchtime approaches once again, and we stick with our routine. Keep the meals balanced and have your snacks handy for the eight-hour window.

Evening. The third evening will be similar to the second and subsequent evenings. You have your dinner and desired snacks, but nothing past seven PM except water.

Key Points:

- Be mindful and take notes.
- Stay with your determined eating patterns.
- Stay hydrated.

Thursday (Day 4)

Morning. Similar to previous days, be mindful of your awakening and take note of any feelings, positive or negative. Keep hydrated and be appreciative and excited for your eating window.

Midday. The beginning of the eating window on this day is a milestone. You are halfway through the first week, and the practice is becoming comfortable and not unlike any other routine before you discovered fasting. Have your standard lunch and snacks. Be mindful and smile!

Evening. Trekking on through the halfway point, this night is much like the previous ones – a nice dinner and halt your caloric intake at seven PM. This evening is a good one to note any differences in your sleeping patterns. Are you falling asleep more easily? Are you sleeping through the night?

Key Points:

- Stay mindful and take notes.
- Contemplate the halfway mark.
- Stay within your eating patterns.
- Stay hydrated.

Friday (Day 5)

Morning. TGIF and another beautiful morning as usual. Be mindful and aware, stay hydrated, and continue with your day until eleven AM when you get to enjoy some food.

Midday. Eleven AM rolls around, and it's time for a snack or meal. Enjoy and take notes of any excitement you feel about your first weekend of fasting. Eat as you wish and stay hydrated.

Evening. The evening approaches and many people are taking advantage of the weekend – going out for drinks and music, etc. You have your allotted time for eating, so if you enjoy an alcoholic drink sometimes, feel free to have one but not after seven PM. (Of course, if you feel comfortable, you can intake calories past seven PM, but be sure to keep track of the time you intake your last calories and adjust the time for Saturday accordingly.)

Key Points:
- Stay mindful and take notes.
- Stay within eating patterns.
- Consider alcohol and social life and how it can affect the patterns.
- Stay hydrated. (optional)

Saturday (Day 6)

Morning. Your first weekend morning with the new fast and all is well. You may have the day off today and find yourself trying to fill the time since you are not preparing and planning as much food as usual. This morning is a great time to think about adding an exercise routine or explore other changes you may want to make for next week.

Midday. A free day is a great time to have a hike or run errands to fill time. Take note of whether or not the fasting has affected minuscule tasks like grocery shopping. Do the foods at the store seem more or less appealing? Are you less stressed while running errands or spending time in the car? A day off is a great time to really analyze the subtle transformation that is taking place. Keep your routine and only intake calories during a predetermined time slot.

Evening. The day off is coming to a close, and you have some dinner and perhaps a drink to ease into the night. This evening will seem especially exciting as you enter into Sunday and start your second week.

Key Points:

- Be aware and mindful, and don't forget to take notes.
- Consider days off and the extra free time you have.
- Stay hydrated.

Sunday (Day 7)

Whether your eighth day falls on a Sunday or not, this day is good to reflect on the past week. Look over any notes you've taken mentally or physically and see if you want to make any changes for the upcoming week. Keep your eating schedule during this time as well, although fun customization for this day could be what is known as a 'cheat' day, where you ignore you fasting practice and eat whenever you like. Another form of a cheat day would be simply to eliminate the exercise portion of the day. For our purposes of weight loss and transformation, we will stick with our routine and practice, so the eating window remains from eleven AM to seven PM.

You have completed your first official week of IF using the 16/8 method! For the following weeks, you can continue to keep up this pattern or even customize or switch to a different method. Always remember: this is your practice to improve your life. Make it your own and continue to keep notes on your progress and feelings. Don't be afraid to feel proud and accomplished with your new routine. Share the joys with coworkers and friends, and most importantly, enjoy the new and ever-changing you!

The 5/2 Method

As we discussed earlier, this method looks more like a diet than a fast, but instead of restricting certain foods, you are restricting the time frame in which you enjoy these foods. The 5/2 method involves having meals as you typically would but choosing two days of the week to consume less than 600 calories for the entire day. For this seven-day guideline, we will approach it as a standard work week, with Saturdays and Sundays as the days off.

Sunday

We start our guide on Sunday to take time to prepare for the upcoming week. Today, you should make sure you are stocked up on groceries and have the next seven days loosely scheduled. Prepping the meals for the calorie-restricted days is an excellent way to control caloric intake. Some questions of whether or not you need to make dietary changes or add some physical activity to your normal routine: *Is my typical diet nutrient-rich? Do I stay hydrated throughout the day? How much exercise do I get each week?* These questions will help alter and optimize your fasting experience. You also need to choose which two days of the week you are going to restrict caloric intake. These two days can be together like Tuesday-Wednesday or a day or two apart, such as Tuesday and Thursday, which will be the days we choose for this guide. Exercise for this guide, in particular, will be performed in the morning. Take time today to be mindful of the upcoming week and take notes of your feelings and experiences going into this new routine.

Monday (Day 1)

You awake to your first week on the 5/2 method to business as usual. Treat this day like any other; you can eat how you typically do, exercise as you normally do, and go about your day. If you feel that you have an unhealthy diet, then switching to some more nutrient dense foods will only help this process. And likewise, if you do not typically exercise, then adding some light stretching or a short walk in the morning is a good idea. If you feel that you do not ingest enough water, now is a great time to start being stricter on hydration; otherwise, this would be just a normal Monday. Be aware and mindful of how you are feeling today and take note of any new experiences the changes you make to your routine may bring.

Once the evening comes, prepare your mind and body for your first calorie-restricted day tomorrow, also your 600 calories for that day. Whether you're choosing two small meals or to snack throughout the day, have them prepared so that you will not need to worry about it tomorrow. For this guide, we will be choosing two small meals. Also, keep in mind that the transition from a typical day to restricted day will be easier the more similar the diets are day to day. For example, eating 4,000 calories today then only 600 tomorrow will be a much tougher transition than a calorie count that is closer to an average amount, around 2,000 calories.

Tuesday (Day 2)

You awake on your first calorie-restricted day. Take note on how your mindset will be: are you confident in your ability to succeed? Are you excited for this new journey? Taking notes to compare to future mornings is highly recommended. So, you start your day by drinking plenty of water, some light exercise of your choosing, and you will opt out of breakfast today.

Once lunchtime approaches, you can enjoy one of your small 300-calorie meals or snacks. Be aware of how enjoyable such a small meal can be: are you excited about this meal even knowing it's small and there's not much more to come? Is the small amount discouraging? Although it's not as much as you're used to, your body knows something is new and will adapt. Have plenty of water if you do not feel full and continue with the day.

The evening approaches, and it's time for another meal. Are you excited for this meal? Do you feel hungry? Analyze this first dinner and be truthful with yourself. You may desire more food but be strong and fill up on water or perhaps some non-caffeinated tea or coffee. Take note of similar experiences for bedtime: are you falling asleep easier? Are you thinking about more food? Be reassured that tomorrow is a normal day and you can eat what you like.

Wednesday (Day 3)

Another normal day as you arise. Before you hit the kitchen for breakfast, take note of how you feel and perhaps contemplate it over your light morning exercise. Now, you can have a meal as per usual and go about your day, periodically stopping and taking the time to be mindful and aware of any new experiences.

This day will continue like a typical day. In the evening, be sure to have your 600 calories planned out for tomorrow, and again, be aware of your bedtime experiences.

Thursday (Day 4)

Your second morning of calorie-restricted intake is a milestone. You have made it halfway through the first week of your new life. This day will be identical to Tuesday (Day 2) as you will be having two 300-calorie meals. Of course, if you wish to change the time of the day, you have your meals, and that's fine. For this guide, we will stick with exercise this morning with plenty of water and an optional non-caloric drink (coffee, tea) but no meal until lunch.

Lunchtime approaches and you're ready for the meal. Enjoy it and be aware of how this new routine makes you feel. Be mindful of the flavors and ask yourself similar questions just like Tuesday.

The evening approaches and you see your second meal in the near future. Be aware of your feelings leading up to the meal and continue being aware of any new experiences. Treat bedtime the same with mindfulness and awareness.

Friday (Day 5)

Today, you awake and treat it like the previous mornings – exercise, hydration, and mindfulness. However, you get to eat normally, so enjoy breakfast and lunch accordingly.

Once the evening comes, you are aware that weekends are spent relaxing, maybe with alcoholic drinks and socializing. This is permitted since today is not a restricted day.

Saturday (Day 6)

This day is similar to yesterday. Although it is a day off and you have no restrictions on caloric intake, continue being mindful of your new routine: *Do I want to change or intensify next week's practice? Do I feel comfortable with the new routine?* Spend this day off as you normally would but with your new lifestyle in the back of your mind.

Sunday (Day 7)

This is the final day of the seven-day week. Treat this day as you would any – no calorie restriction or boundaries, just a basic day off before the work week begins again. Did you decide to alter the routine from last week? If so, make sure you have meals prepared and have the schedule all worked out for your upcoming second week with the 5/2 method.

Upon completion of the first week, what subtle changes have you seen in yourself and body? Do you feel that this week was a success? Take a deep breath and congratulate yourself on a new journey, and make a commitment to stay on a mindful path for the foreseeable future.

The Eat Stop Eat Method

This method of IF is a little more taxing on the body as it requires a full 24-hour fast one or two times a week. The fast itself asks you not to consume any calories for a full 24 hours. So, essentially, the only thing you will ingest is water. Non-caloric drinks are acceptable as well, such as coffee and tea. The non-caloric drinks should not have milk or sugar added to them and also be aware of caffeine content in these drinks, especially with an empty stomach. And since this method is slightly more intensive, you need to be even more cautious as a beginner approaching this style of fasting.

Sunday

While preparing for the 'eat stop eat' method, you need to take a serious look at your previous relationship with fasting and food itself. If you have no previous experience with calorie restriction, it is recommended that you experiment with it, perhaps with one of the other methods in this book, to make sure you are comfortable with a full day of no calorie intake. It is also important that when you are having meals during the next seven days that you eat food that your body is used to having. Eat your usual diet and similar foods. With this caution on your mind, you can proceed to prepare your upcoming week.

So today, your responsibilities include preparing your mind and body for the upcoming week of IF. Going without calories for 24 hours is something your body has generally not experienced your whole life, but be reminded that it can be safely practiced and has been safely practiced for centuries. First of all, you need to decide the day(s) that you are choosing to fast on. For this guide, we will be fasting for two days out of the week, Tuesday (Day 2) and Thursday (Day 4). These days, of course, can be changed at your convenience and preference. Once you have selected your days, contemplate and plan your days.

While considering your next week, you need to take into consideration your diet. If you have a poor diet, then it may be a good idea to change your diet to the guidelines in the previous chapter for a week or two before the IF begins. Although you are fasting on only two days, the week itself should still be viewed as a part of the fasting practice. You need to make sure you have your proper groceries and plenty of water. To optimize the week, you can even meal prep and prepare your meals for each day and have them ready to go in the refrigerator or other storage. Remain mindful and listen to your body. As you spend this day like any other, you will keep the beginning of your transformational week in mind well into the evening and off to bed.

Monday (Day 1)

Luckily, for one of the more intensive fasts in this book, the eat stop eat method requires you to eat precisely what you would normally eat on non-fast days. This fast asks that you do not dramatically alter your normal eating schedule on the non-fast days as to avoid putting too much strain and change on your body in such a short amount of time. This will make the non-fasting days pretty simple, but you also need to maintain your awareness and mindfulness throughout the week even on days when you can eat. And so, for Monday, simply go about your day as usual while ensuring your mind is prepared for the calorie-restricted day tomorrow. It is recommended to eat on the lighter side of your normal diet tonight and, of course, keep very hydrated.

Tuesday (Day 2)

You awake on your first full fast day mentally prepared and ready to take on this new practice. Taking plenty of water first thing in the morning and accompanying some light exercise is ideal. If you must have caffeine in the morning, the acceptable drinks are coffee and tea as long as it is not sweetened or mixed with other additives. Regardless of how you spend your day, you need to be sure that you have access to plenty of water throughout the day. Consistently drink water, but don't consume it too quickly.

This is the plan for the entire day. No calories, just water. As simple as it is, you may be craving food as your body is used to meals at certain times. This may be uncomfortable, at first, but stay busy and keep in mind that you are trying to reset your body's rhythms. One aspect of the completely restricted day is all the free time you have. If you're working on this day, it may not be as noticeable. However, once you arrive home, there will be plenty of free time. Try to stay busy by having planned activities to do; a casual walk, household chores, games, and media come in handy with the extra time not spent preparing and cooking meals.

As evening falls and you prepare for sleep, look back on your first fast day and analyze your experiences: did the lack of food aggravate you? How do you feel physically? Do things seem altered in some way? These questions help to keep track of your experiences and recall them for comparison later after your second fast day. If you have trouble falling asleep, a book or light stretching helps greatly.

Wednesday (Day 3)

The third day of your IF week will be very similar to the first. But when you first awake, be conscious of how you feel with such an empty stomach: is it difficult or easier to get out of bed? Do you feel lighter? Are you terribly eager to have some food? Start the day with light exercise and water and eat as you normally would – having a similar calorie intake as the first day of this week. Take note of how the food tastes and how it feels entering your body after a day of no eating. This day will continue as normal with mindfulness and awareness of your next fast day.

Thursday (Day 4)

Your second and final fully restricted day of the week is upon you. Much like Day 2, you will begin with plenty of water and light exercise in the morning, optional caffeinated non-caloric drinks, and mindfulness. Again, consistently take note of your experiences and feelings. This day shouldn't be any more difficult than the first calorie-restricted day – since you have a general idea of what to expect. As such, you will have access to plenty of water and keep hydrated throughout the day, paying attention to your experiences and staying busy.

As the evening approaches, you will spend the time keeping your mind occupied and preparing for a full night's sleep.

Friday (Day 5)

This day will begin similar to Day 3 in that you will take note of how you feel in the morning and how waking with an empty stomach affects you physically and mentally. You have completed your calorie-restricted days for the week, but keep your experiences fresh on your mind and contemplate them over the weekend. Today and the next, you will be on your regular eating schedule as well.

Saturday (Day 6)

This day will be identical to yesterday, and you will remain on your normal eating schedule. Today, you will also decide if you want to keep your same IF regimen for next week. Taking into consideration all your experiences from the past six days, you need to ask yourself: *was this week a success? Will I keep this Intermittent Fasting method for the upcoming week or try a different approach? Did the days I chose to fast fit my schedule conveniently?* Once you have answered these questions, you can go about your day as usual.

Sunday (Day 7)

Now, you have hit Day 7, and you should have a general idea of what you want to do as far as fasting is concerned for the next seven days. You will prepare for the upcoming week accordingly and ensure you have the proper supplies and schedule.

Added Notes on the Eat Stop Eat Method

Having explored this method of IF thoroughly, you can alter this method in many ways. One way to step up the intensity of the practice is to push the calorie-restricted days together and go an entire 48 hours without the caloric intake. Not only is this a great way to ensure the body uses reserved fat energy, but it is also a great test of the mind and your commitment to your transformation. The two days together is not recommended for beginners and will require much thought and dedication to yourself and this respected practice.

Alternate Day Method

The alternate day method requires that you alternate your fast days every other day – that is if you didn't restrict calories today, then tomorrow you are to restrict calories in some manner. This method is great to customize for your practice. For our guide here, we will be borrowing from the 5/2 diet and cut back your calorie intake to less than 600 calories on fasting days. You will approach this method in the guide as a standard work week with Saturday and Sundays being days off, but, of course, synchronize this practice up with your schedule accordingly. In this guide, your first restricted day will be Tuesday.

Sunday

As with the previous guides, you will begin with the day before your first official day to contemplate and prepare for the upcoming week. You need to make sure you have plenty of groceries and access to water and that you are mentally prepared for the practice you're about to commit to. Prepping meals works great for this method as you can prepare a meal with the desired number of calories beforehand and have them ready to go in the refrigerator. This helps to control your calorie intake and allows you not to have to worry about preparing food throughout the week as you navigate the IF terrain. As you prepare for this week, be mindful and aware of what you are committing to and get plenty of rest tonight.

Monday (Day 1)

Today will be like any normal day. You will wake up and have your standard morning routine. If exercise isn't a part of this routine, this week is a good time to add it in. Plenty of water as needed and you will go about your day, and as usual, keeping in mind that tomorrow is a restricted intake day. If you are changing your diet as well this week, this method asks that you do not dramatically alter your non-fast days too wildly, but adding nutrient-rich foods is always a good idea regardless of what week it is. Having another normal day complete, you spend the evening mentally preparing for tomorrow, keeping note of your experiences and anticipation.

Tuesday (Day 2)

Morning. Your first restricted intake day begins as you awake. Plenty of water and light exercise is on the agenda for the morning. Coffee and tea are acceptable, but be aware of any calories you're adding with sugars and milk as you are only ingesting around 600 calories today in a two-meal approach. Contemplate your experience this morning: *am I excited about my new practice? Do I feel that my new routine is in sync with the rest of my life?* You complete your morning and move along to lunchtime.

Midday. As midday approaches, you can have your first 300-calorie meal for the day. As you begin the meal, analyze your experience: *is this a satisfying amount of food? Did I make proper choices for the contents of this meal? How does this experience differ from other lunches in my recent past?* You complete lunch and continue with your day as usual, being aware of how your body feels and staying hydrated.

Evening. Once nightfall approaches, you can enjoy your dinner, another 300-calorie meal comprised of nutrient-dense foods loosely based on the guidelines in Chapter 6. With this meal, you near the end of your first calorie-restricted day. Think about your experience: *what were the hours in between meals like? Am I still craving food after this evening meal? How enjoyable was the food with such restricted intake*? With bedtime approaching, focus on your mind and body, keeping note of any feelings or experiences as you fall asleep.

Wednesday (Day 3)

This morning will be like Day 1, although you are waking up to a calorie-restricted body. You will have plenty of water and light exercise, then continue your day with a normal intake of food and drink while keeping consistent attention to any new experiences and feelings. You stay aware that tomorrow is a restricted intake day and you should consider yesterday: *were the meals up to par? Could I slightly alter tomorrow to optimize my practice?* Feel free to customize as you wish; this is your IF practice.

Thursday (Day 4)

This day will be identical to Day 2 unless you decide to make any changes. For this guide, we will keep to your set guidelines and treat this day the same as Day 2 – water and light exercise in the morning, a 300-calorie meal for lunch, and a 300-calorie meal for dinner. All the while taking note of your experiences and being mindful of your changes.

Friday (Day 5)

Similar to Days 1 and 3, Day 5 is a day to go about your normal eating schedule. Spend the day on your regular schedule and eat meals similar to Days 1 and 3. As you continue to alternate days, be aware of how the practice differs on calorie-restricted days: *how was Day 1 different from Day 5? Has calorie restriction become easier to practice? How are my energy levels?* By comparing the days and actively engaging with the experiences, you can get a firm grip on how you want your IF practice to evolve.

Saturday (Day 6)

As a day that is not a calorie-restricted day, you will go about your business as usual, eating meals similar to Days 2 and 4, maintaining awareness of your IF even on this non-fast day. As you can see, the alternating day method allows you to maintain a nice pattern that is easy to keep track of. This method is noticeably great for beginners with its easy to follow guidelines and excellent flexibility. Treat this day as a celebratory one as well as you near the end of your first week of IF. Perhaps treat yourself to a sweet treat or a night out with friends.

Sunday (Day 7)

Today is a calorie-restricted day to be treated like Days 1, 3, and 5. The morning is spent drinking water and some light exercise.

Lunch is a 300-calorie nutrient-rich meal, and dinner is also a 300-calorie nutrient-rich meal.

You must also decide if you are going to continue this pattern for the upcoming week. If you find that this practice is working, then you will continue alternating days for the next week or even month! Keeping this pattern solid for many weeks will inevitably lead to this diet being your normal practice and seem like any other day compared to the days that filled this past week. Customize as you wish and, of course, always stay mindful and aware of what your body is telling you.

Warrior Method

Our next method is the warrior method. Named in regards to Paleo diets and warrior tribes of ancient man, this method calls for meals that are as raw and unprocessed as possible. If your diet is not in line with this guideline, it may help to adhere to a Paleo-like diet the week before beginning this method.

The warrior method is a relatively simple one to follow as it does not require any days that are one hundred percent calorie-restricted. This method of IF involves one huge meal in the evening time while simply eating raw and unprocessed snacks throughout the day or just no calories throughout the day. For our guide in this book, you will casually snack during the day and have a big nutrient-rich meal in the evening. You will treat the upcoming week as a typical work week with a standard weekend.

Sunday

The day before you begin your warrior fast, you need to spend the day preparing your body and mind for the changes and new routine you are approaching this week. Ensure that you have plenty of unprocessed snack foods readily available; nuts, fruits, and veggies are ideal for the daytime snacking. Access to plenty of water and a general idea of what you wish to have for large evening meals is a must. As you get ready for bed, consider your ancient ancestors and their very raw, unprocessed diet. Also, maintain your mindful and confident approach to this new routine of IF.

Monday (Day 1)

Daytime. The first day of your method will be started with plenty of water and light exercise. As mentioned, you will be snacking throughout the day, so you may enjoy your raw foods as you wish. For this guide, you will be having a very light breakfast of raw foods and perhaps a tea or coffee as well. As the day rolls on, you can have tiny amounts of nuts and berries throughout, being cautious not to eat a whole day's worth of snacks in one sitting.

As lunchtime approaches, maintain this mentality – only having snacks here and there through the day. Be mindful of the experiences you face: are you craving the other snacks you've prepared? Are you having a hard time not eating all your supplies? How would tiny snacks compare to no food at all?

Nighttime. The evening approaches, and you can start considering your first big meal of the week. Preparing it should require minimal cooking, so feel free to be creative. Steaming foods instead of frying is a great way to stay in line with these guidelines. This meal can be whatever you wish but stay within the structure of the least processed foods – no frozen meals, no fast foods, and no deep frying. Avoiding as much prepackaged food as possible is key. With this in mind, there is an upside that this meal is meant to be huge. Feel free to fill your belly nice and full of nutrient-rich foods this evening. Keep a note on how your body reacts to this: do you feel full more quickly or with less food than usual? Is raw food as enjoyable as your normal choices for dinner? Note these experiences as you are going to compare each evening's experiences as you move through the week. It helps to have similar meals through this week as well, but it's not mandatory.

Tuesday (Day 2)

Daytime. The second day and all subsequent days for that matter are very similar to Day 1. This method requires consistency and a real focus on how raw your foods are, which has not been an issue for the previous methods in this book. With this in mind, you start Day 2 just like Day 1; plenty of water, light exercise, and if you so choose, a very light raw snack, preferably fruits, veggies, and nuts. On with the day, you continue to snack. Compare this day to yesterday: *do I feel any different? Am I adapting easily to only having raw snacks during the day?* Keep a close watch on how your day-to-day experience changes subtly as you continue the warrior method.

Nighttime. This evening will be very similar to last night. Prepare a large meal as unprocessed as possible and as nutrient-rich as possible. Although the evenings like this are going to repeat, be very aware of any changes in your experience and relationship with the larger meals: *am I excited to enjoy this meal? How have I adapted to the new raw diet?* Continue this evaluation consistently through the week every night before and after the meal.

Wednesday (Day 3)

Daytime. As mentioned earlier, this method is about consistency and maintaining an unprocessed diet. So naturally, Day 3 looks identical to the previous days; plenty of water and light exercise in the morning, snacking lightly on raw foods throughout the day, and the ever-important mindfulness and awareness as you see subtle changes in your mind and body.

Nighttime. Another similar night approaches and you anticipate another unprocessed meal. Keeping the large meal similar in caloric intake and size, you move onward on your warrior journey, keeping note of those subtle changes and experiences each day.

Thursday (Day 4)

Daytime. Day 4 is like any other during this repetitious week: water and exercise fill the morning and raw snacking all day in tiny amounts. By this time in the week, the changes may be less subtle as your body adapts into its new routine. Continue the process, confident and aware.

Nighttime. This evening is like the previous ones. If you feel a little bored of the similar meals, always remember that this is your practice and you can customize as you like. Just try your hardest not to venture too far outside of the structures and patterns that you have established.

Friday (Day 5)

Daytime. Another morning of hydration and light exercise. You've made it one work week, so how are you feeling? Are there any noticeable changes physically or mentally? Continue your snacking guidelines and keep the mindfulness at the forefront of your thoughts.

Nighttime. This evening is just like the others, but it is the weekend, so maybe reward your dedication with a night out for drinks or socializing to break up the monotony of this method. Maintain your awareness and see if there are any new changes in the way you view a social setting or a casual glass of wine at home.

Saturday (Day 6)

Daytime. Day 6 remains unchanged compared to the previous days. It is a weekend, so if you wish, you can skip exercise, but plenty of water and keep on snacking as per usual. At this point, the patterns should seem pretty set into place in your mind and body, but take this day to look back on the week: *is the warrior method working for my lifestyle? How has my mind and body changed in just one week? Is this new practice creating new paths in my day-to-day life?*

Consider if you wish to continue this method for next week and take your time as you analyze the past six days.

Nighttime. Time for another large meal, again maintaining the structure and guidelines as much as possible. Once bedtime approaches, you should have a firm grasp on whether or not you are continuing this method or any other changes coming for next week.

Sunday (Day 7)

You have managed to keep your IF protocol under control for a full week now. How different do you feel compared to seven days ago? You will still treat this day as a warrior fast day but will take action in making necessary adjustments for the upcoming week. Any groceries or other suitable supplies need to be available, and you should be aware of any alterations you are making this week. Perhaps you wish to change your snacking options? Maybe you need a 'cheat' day once a week for now? All the possible customizations are endless as you analyze your needs and desires. With that in mind, you approach another large meal and can start implementing your changes as soon as you wish or simply keep going with your established patterns for as many weeks as you like.

Spontaneity Method

We now move on to our final example of IF methods. The spontaneity method is pretty self-explanatory: you may spontaneously choose when to fast as you see fit. Not feeling hungry today? Restrict calories. Feel like only eating raw foods today? Make it happen. Simply want to cut out sweets for a week? Easy. The endless possibilities with this method make it great for beginners who wish to experiment with different methods to see what feels right. It also works for busy people and parents who want to keep a mindful approach to health but don't have the schedule to adhere to strict guidelines and rules. And sure, this may seem like you're only skipping meals because it's convenient or a lazy way to fast, but if we can funnel our perception of our diets and lifestyles through an 'intermittent fasting lens' by maintaining mindfulness and awareness about our bodies and how fasting affects them, then we will find that a spontaneous method can work just as well as any other. To reiterate, no one way works for everyone, and some people thrive under less structured conditions.

For this method, you will not require a day-by-day guide since that would contradict the purpose of spontaneity. You will, however, explore some ideas and suggestions for this method.

Being spontaneous can have an amazing effect on the mind. It adds a sense of freedom to a monotonous week or month and can really help people relax and live in the moment. When it comes to fasting, it works the same way. Go with your gut; if you feel strongly about just eating some delicious fruit all day, do it and call it a part of your fasting routine. Often, when this practice is put into play seriously, use a pattern, and structure forms in itself, and the practitioner finds themselves having a solid IF routine without even trying to. While also taking ideas from the previously mentioned methods, here are some ideas to throw into your spontaneous practice:

- Go with your gut; if you feel it, do it.
- 24-hour calorie restriction. Waking up feeling like a day fast? Make it happen.
- Not hungry when you wake up? Skip breakfast and/or lunch.
- Feel like you've had too much sugar lately? Cut out sweets or alcohol for a set duration of time.
- Blink and the day has flown by without food? Call it a fast and go to bed.
- Does your religion or spiritual preference have a holiday that traditionally requires fasting? Try it out.

The list could go forever, but keep in mind the serious nature of fasting and always approach it with your overall wellbeing in mind. You can take this method and make your own rules but always accompany these rules with research and contemplation. Also, it is good to state that although this method is a free form, it is not particularly a good idea to use the easy-going nature of this fast as an excuse not to stay with your convictions. If you state to yourself that you are fasting or planning to, stick with it. Commitment and dedication are two of the most important factors and lessons of IF.

We have officially explored some of the more popular methods of Intermittent Fasting. These guidelines will act as a great stepping stone to your customized methods if you decide to stay with the IF lifestyle. As you continue on this journey, always maintain mindfulness and awareness about your body and mind.

Chapter 9: Dos and Don'ts of Intermittent Fasting

All the myths and broad array of opinions about the subject can make fasting research a nightmare on the Internet, but don't be disheartened by people online and stay focused on your goals. This doesn't mean to go headfirst into it without being aware of the dangers that can come with a haphazard practice. Keeping a keen eye out for red flags from your body is important. Safety is overall the most important thing when it comes to these transformative practices and, of course, we're trying to improve our health not destroy it.

The following list will serve as a quick reference guide to safe Intermittent Fasting. If you have any doubts or questions that remain unanswered in this book, the following guide should give insight and act as a general basis for the unwritten rules of fasting. With all the information we have explored throughout this book, you should be readily prepared to begin an IF regimen, but, as with anything in life, there can be unexpected twists and turns. If there are any doubts in your mind, expand your research or consult your physician for advice. And, as always, your body knows best; do what feels right but also consider this list.

Do make sure you are fit to fast. There are plenty of physical conditions that should not be combined with IF. You should not be fasting if:

- You are pregnant or lactating.
- You have diabetes.
- You are under the age of eighteen.
- You have a serious medical condition.
- You are taking prescription drugs that may have unpredictable results while fasting.

Do let your friends and family know you are fasting. Not only is spending time with friends and family a great way to spend downtime during a fast but having their support will also help you attain your goals. Be sure to let them know all about fasting if they are not familiar with the practice. This can help the uninformed understand the practice so that they don't think you're starving yourself. Also, in some cases, your friends and family may be interested in starting an IF practice themselves and having a fasting partner just makes it a little easier.

Do let your primary care provider know that you are interested in fasting. He or she will need to know this to customize their approach to treating you. The transformative nature of IF should be handled with great care, and your doctor, knowing this information, will be key to optimizing the effects of the fast.

Do take vitamins as needed. Depending on the method of fasting you choose, you may feel the need to supplement your vitamins and minerals. Since you're cutting back on the amount of food you're consuming, you may need a little extra help replacing some nutrients you would normally rely on. It is not mandatory to supplement; it's not for everyone, but it is safe to do so. Most certainly consult your physician if you have other questions about the supplements.

Do prepare your mind and body. We stress this a lot throughout the book, but it is a very important point that needs to be addressed. By asking yourself tough questions like, "Am I ready to dedicate myself to this fast?" will allow you to see what needs to be done to prepare yourself for the fast. Actively thinking about your intentions and goals goes a long way to analyze your lifestyle and what you want to get out of an IF practice. Meditation, yoga, and improving your diet during the weeks leading up to the fast are only going to help you ease into the transformation.

Do prepare your home. If your home is full of junk food and other tempting things that could jeopardize your success, it is recommended that you rid yourself of these things. This is not only a practice in maintaining self-control but of also cleansing your house of your past. This is a part of the transformation process and does wonders to make your home feel spacious and uncluttered. Maybe rearrange your furniture the way you intend to rearrange your health. Hang positive and welcoming décor, and overall, let your surrounding change with you.

Do plan your fasting days. You want to make sure that the week(s) you choose to fast are ones that will be relatively stress-free and not the busiest week/s of the year. Planning a fast during a holiday that involves sweets and feasts is setting yourself up for failure. Planning a fast during a marathon you intend to run is just asking for trouble. Ensure there are no major events that will hinder your focus on attaining your goals with IF.

Do have fun. Be proud that you're taking control of your health with IF. You will come across skeptics and critics, but stay focused on what you need. This is your practice; it is a part of you, and it aims to improve your overall quality of life. Be confident. Be happy. Be yourself.

Don't forget about water. It's no secret how important water is to everyday living, but during a fast, it is even more important. Staying hydrated should be at the forefront of your mind through the entire fast. This mentality should carry over into everyday life. Drink water. Easy.

Don't stress out. You've probably heard of the slang term 'hangry'. It's used to describe being angry because you're hungry. Although not the most scientific of terms, going without our normal food intake can sometimes lead to stress. Through the stress, many undesired and misunderstood emotions can come through leading to a vicious cycle. When you feel stressed, take five to ten deep breaths or, if possible, walk it off around the block. Your body will get used to the calorie restriction, and these sudden stressors will subside.

Don't overindulge the night before a fast. Depending on the fasting method, it is safe to say that stuffing yourself full of food the night before a fast is counterintuitive. Stuffing your stomach contradicts the entire goal of this practice – developing awareness about your body and shedding excess fat. Try to balance out your mindset a bit by preparing your body for the fast by eating light the night before.

Don't celebrate the end of your fast by overindulging. You may feel starved after a fasting week, but that's no reason to go out drinking heavily or indulging in fried foods. Sure, a treat here and there won't hurt, but don't use your fasting practice as an excuse to be unhealthy. This attitude will build a toxic relationship with your fasting routine. If you want to get a little crazy, do so because you're a little crazy, not because you finished a fast. This potentially can send you right back to where you began.

Don't be afraid to stop your fast. If you find yourself feeling ill or other discomforts during a fast, cut it short. Your health is what is most important, so take any measures possible to avoid harm. It may feel like a defeat, but you can try again in the near future once the issue is resolved. There's no sense is risking great harm just because you want to finish a fast.

This list may not cover all the experiences you will encounter on your journey, but we did touch base on many common mistakes and important things that often get overlooked. Be sure always to consider all the possible outcomes when planning a fast; this is why we put so much emphasis on contemplating and analyzing our experiences while we practice intermittent fasting. Overall the most important aspect of these awareness-enhancing practices is to listen to your body. If you feel more discomfort or especially pain, don't hesitate to postpone your fast until a later date. Consulting your physician is recommended if you experience any concerning pain or discomfort.

Conclusion

Thank you for making it through to the end of *Intermittent Fasting for Women: An Essential Guide to Weight Loss, Fat-Burning, and Healing Your Body Without Sacrificing All Your Favorite Foods*. It should have been informative and provided you with all of the tools you need to achieve your goals – whatever they might be.

As we come to a close, we hope you are feeling prepared for the transformative process that is about to begin. There is much related content about this kind of fasting out in the world and surely more to come as its popularity grows, but this comprehensive book serves as an unbiased and welcoming breath of fresh air in the world of Intermittent Fasting.

A simple glance at the history of Intermittent Fasting and the incredible impact it has had on our world and culture is very evident. As far back into our past as we can see, humans have implemented fasting into their culture for a variety of reasons. Spiritual and religious endeavors use fasting rituals and practices as a means of devotion and insight into the unknown realms that humans have considered since the dawn of time. Fasting has been used as a means to ensure survival in many cultures after food harvests were depleted, leading to long-lived societies yielding residents that are living examples of longevity and health. Right up to the present day, fasting remains a staple in indigenous cultures and technologically advantageous societies alike.

As scientists continue to study the effects of Intermittent Fasting on the body and brain, they confirm the value of this amazing practice and solidify its role as a positive health practice whose benefits are seemingly endless. As we conclude this book and continue with our personal practice, we keep in mind the history, influence, and newfound scientific backing that validates Intermittent Fasting as a legitimate, beneficial health practice. The foundation that Intermittent Fasting has built for itself is one that is unshakeable as it moves swiftly into the mainstream culture of the Western world.

As you achieve your goals with these methods, the next step is to continue with your routine, changing it as your life changes, transforming with it as it is a part of you now. Keeping a journal on your experiences comes in handy too – see your progress and be proud, feel accomplished, and live to the fullest. Sharing your experience with others can also be important; sometimes, the only thing someone needs to start their journey is a personal friend to discuss and inform them of the wonders of the Intermittent Fasting lifestyle.

Finally, if you found this book useful in any way, a review on Amazon is always appreciated!

Check out more books by Elizabeth Moore

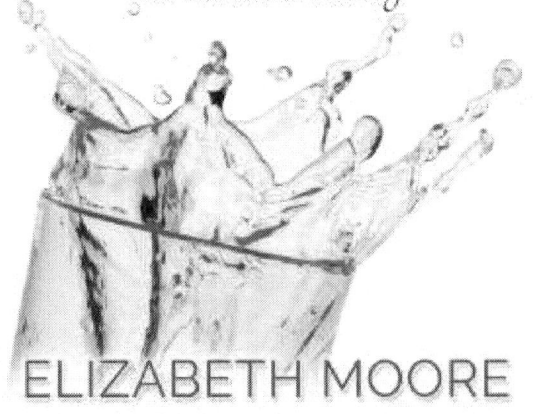

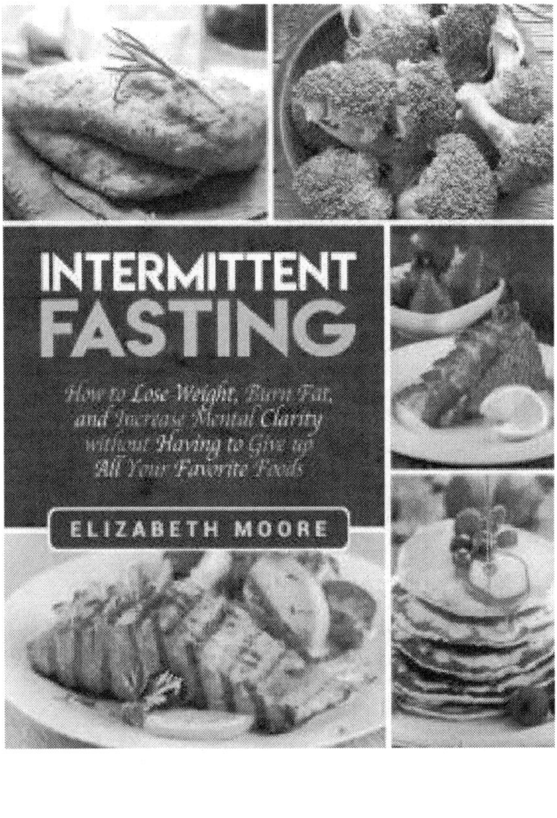
INTERMITTENT
FASTING
How to Lose Weight, Burn Fat,
and Increase Mental Clarity
without Having to Give up
All Your Favorite Foods
ELIZABETH MOORE

AUTOPHAGY

UNLOCK THE SECRETS OF WEIGHT LOSS, ANTI-AGING, AND HEALING WITH INTERMITTENT AND EXTENDED WATER FASTING

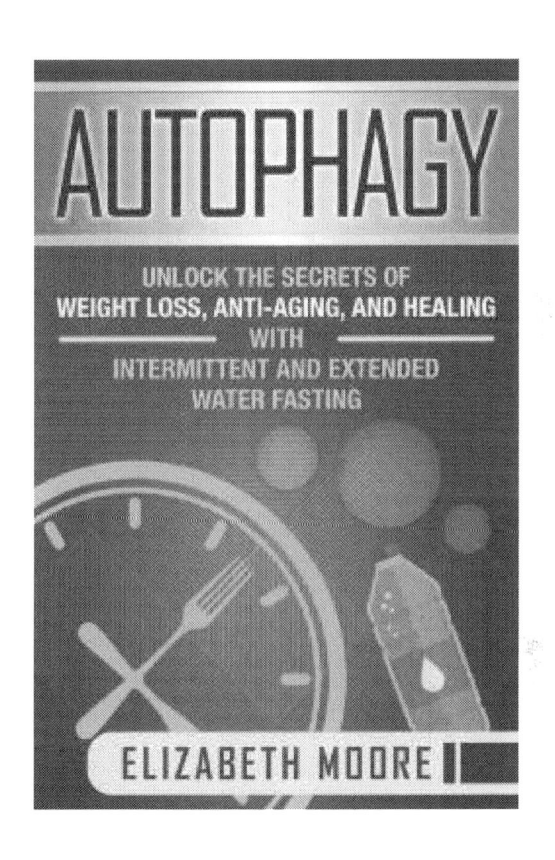

ELIZABETH MOORE

Printed in Great Britain
by Amazon